MW01697711

PEARSON

ALWAYS LEARNING

Jane Rice, RN, CMA-C

Medical Terminology for Health Care Professionals Workbook Pages for the 9th Edition

Custom Edition

Taken from:
Medical Terminology for Health Care Professionals, Ninth Edition
by Jane Rice

Taken from:

Medical Terminology for Health Care Professionals, Ninth Edition
by Jane Rice

This special edition published in cooperation with Pearson Education, Inc.

Pearson Education, Inc., 330 Hudson Street, New York, New York 10013
A Pearson Education Company
www.pearsoned.com

Printed in the United States of America

000200010272143850

CC

PEARSON

ISBN 10: 1-323-83731-0
ISBN 13: 978-1-323-83731-3

CONTENTS IN BRIEF

Study and Review

Word Parts

Prefixes

Give the definitions of the following prefixes.

1. a- ______________________
2. ab- ______________________
3. anti- ______________________
4. cac- ______________________
5. centi- ______________________
6. dia- ______________________
7. hetero- ______________________
8. mal- ______________________
9. micro- ______________________
10. mill- ______________________
11. multi- ______________________
12. para- ______________________

13. pro- ______________________

14. syn- ______________________

15. dis- ______________________

16. epi- ______________________

17. ex- ______________________

18. in- ______________________

Roots and Combining Forms

Give the definitions of the following roots and combining forms.

1. adhes ______________________
2. axill ______________________
3. centr/i ______________________
4. chem/o ______________________
5. format ______________________
6. gene ______________________
7. kil/o ______________________
8. macr/o ______________________
9. necr ______________________
10. norm ______________________
11. onc/o ______________________
12. organ ______________________
13. pyr ______________________
14. pyr/o ______________________
15. radi/o ______________________
16. scop ______________________
17. sept ______________________
18. therm/o ______________________
19. tuss ______________________
20. infect ______________________
21. dem ______________________
22. eti/o ______________________
23. cis ______________________
24. malign ______________________
25. maxim ______________________
26. minim ______________________
27. palm ______________________
28. prophylact ______________________

Suffixes

Give the definitions of the following suffixes.

1. -al ______________________
2. -ary ______________________
3. -centesis ______________________
4. -drome ______________________
5. -form ______________________
6. -genic ______________________
7. -gnosis ______________________
8. -grade ______________________
9. -gram ______________________
10. -hexia ______________________

11. -ic ____________________

12. -ion ____________________

13. -ism ____________________

14. -ive ____________________

15. -liter ____________________

16. -logy ____________________

17. -meter ____________________

18. -osis ____________________

19. -ous ____________________

20. -phoresis ____________________

21. -scope ____________________

22. -sepsis ____________________

23. -therapy ____________________

24. -ar ____________________

Identifying Medical Terms

In the spaces provided, write the medical terms for the following meanings.

1. ____________________ Process of being stuck together
2. ____________________ Without decay
3. ____________________ Pertaining to the armpit
4. ____________________ Use of chemical agents in the treatment of disease
5. ____________________ Pertaining to a different formation
6. ____________________ Process of being badly shaped, deformed
7. ____________________ Scientific instrument designed to view small objects
8. ____________________ Occurring in or having many shapes
9. ____________________ Study of tumors

Matching

Select the appropriate lettered meaning for each of the following words.

_____ 1. abate
_____ 2. antipyretic
_____ 3. cachexia
_____ 4. diagnosis
_____ 5. disease
_____ 6. etiology
_____ 7. illness
_____ 8. prognosis
_____ 9. prophylactic
_____ 10. triage

a. Literally means *lack of ease*
b. State of being sick
c. Pertaining to protecting against disease or pregnancy
d. Pertaining to an agent that is used to lower an elevated body temperature (fever)
e. A system of prioritizing and classifying patient injuries to determine priority of need and treatment
f. To lessen, ease, decrease, or cease
g. Determination of the cause and nature of a disease
h. New disease
i. Literally means *a state of foreknowledge*
j. Condition of ill health, malnutrition, and wasting
k. Study of the cause(s) of disease

Abbreviations

Place the correct word, phrase, or abbreviation in the space provided.

1. CC _____
2. ax _____
3. biopsy _____
4. weight _____
5. Neuro _____
6. ear, nose, throat (otorhinolaryngology) _____
7. dermatology _____
8. gram _____
9. GYN _____
10. Orth _____

Practical Application

Medical Coding

Write your answer to the following questions about terms and abbreviations used in medical coding.

1. Medical coding is the process of assigning __________ characters that represent the diagnoses patients have been given and the services they are to receive.
2. __________ codes identify the reasons that healthcare services were provided.
3. Within the coding system, __________ _____________ is the language used for identifying the diseases and conditions that are coded.
4. The procedure coding system was developed by the ______________________ (CMS) for use in the United States for inpatient hospital settings only.
5. Physicians will continue to use __________________ (CPT) when sending patients for outpatient (OP) testing.

Matching

Select the appropriate lettered meaning for each of the following.

____________	1. HIPAA	a. clinical modification
____________	2. WHO	b. Procedure Coding System
____________	3. CM	c. Health Insurance Portability and Accountability Act
____________	4. PCS	d. Centers for Medicare & Medicaid Services
____________	5. ICD	e. World Health Organization
____________	6. CMS	f. alphabetic characters
____________	7. CPT	g. Centers for Disease Control and Prevention
____________	8. A–Z	h. outpatient
____________	9. OP	i. International Classification of Diseases
____________	10. CDC	j. Current Procedural Terminology

Study and Review

Identifying Suffixes

Underline the suffixes in the following medical words.

1. cardiac	**2.** cephalad	**3.** enuresis	**4.** obstetrician	**5.** bronchiole
6. pustule	**7.** dentalgia	**8.** diabetes	**9.** hyperemesis	**10.** hemoptysis

Defining Suffixes

Give the meaning of the following suffixes.

1. -asthenia ______________________

2. -ion ______________________

3. -itis ______________________

4. -malacia ______________________

5. -megaly ______________________

6. -pathy ______________________

7. -penia ______________________

8. -pepsia ______________________

9. -phobia ______________________

10. -rrhexis ______________________

11. -al ______________________

12. -ar ______________________

13. -ate ______________________

14. -ia ______________________

15. -ize ______________________

16. -oid ______________________

17. -or ______________________

18. -ose ______________________

19. -ous ______________________

20. -um ______________________

Using Suffixes to Build Medical Words

Using a suffix from the following list, build the appropriate medical word.

-al	*-ior*	*-ar*	*-ile*
-ary	*-osis*	*-ia*	*-ula*
-icle	*-us*		

1. Condition of excessive sweating — hyper/hidr/__________

2. Pertaining to muscles — muscul/__________

3. Small spot or discolored area of the skin — mac/__________

4. Condition of loss of hair — a/lopec/__________

5. Literally means *little belly* — ventr/__________

6. Pertaining to a bedsore — de/cubit/__________

7. Pertaining to the skin — integument/__________

8. Pertaining to the penis — pen/__________

9. Pertaining to present at birth — con/genit/__________

10. Pertaining to toward the front of the body — anter/__________

Identifying Medical Terms

In the spaces provided, write the medical terms for the following meanings.

1. ________________________ Process of scraping away from a surface
2. ________________________ To induce a loss of feeling or sensation
3. ________________________ Pertaining to a state of alertness or consciousness
4. ________________________ Unequal in size or shape
5. ________________________ The process whereby a pathogenic organism invades the body and causes disease
6. ________________________ Pertaining to a state of deep sleep
7. ________________________ Refers to the expected resiliency of the skin
8. ________________________ Pertaining to a feeling of greatness
9. ________________________ To resemble a female
10. ________________________ To use the hands or fingers to examine by touch

Practical Application

ICD-10-CM Terminology

Write your answers in the spaces provided.

1. The largest animal phylum that makes up about 85% of all known animals in the world is known as ____________.
2. A ____________ is the scientific way of grouping together related organisms.
3. The term used for the patient having intestinal parasites or worms is ____________
4. A ____________ is a protein-like infectious particle.
5. What is the term that means pertaining to single-celled parasitic organisms with flexible membranes and the ability to move? ____________
6. A ____________ is an organism, such as fleas, mosquitoes, ticks, that transmits a pathogen from one source to another.
7. The term that means pertaining to or containing blood is ____________.
8. The term that is used to describe fungal infections is ____________.
9. The term ____________ means pertaining to spirochetes, especially infections caused by them, such as syphilis.
10. What is the term that means pertaining to inflammation without the production of pus? ____________

Study and Review

Identifying Prefixes

Underline the prefixes in the following medical words.

1. apnea	**2.** bradypnea	**3.** dyspnea	**4.** eupnea	**5.** hyperpnea
6. hypopnea	**7.** tachypnea	**8.** binary	**9.** concentration	**10.** extraocular

Defining Prefixes

Give the meaning of the following prefixes.

1. anti-	______________________	**2.** brachy-	______________________
3. dia-	______________________	**4.** hetero-	______________________
5. homeo-	______________________	**6.** hydro-	______________________
7. micro-	______________________	**8.** oligo-	______________________
9. pan-	______________________	**10.** pseudo-	______________________
11. a-	______________________	**12.** an-	______________________
13. bi-	______________________	**14.** bin-	______________________
15. con-	______________________	**16.** de-	______________________
17. extra-	______________________	**18.** hyper-	______________________
19. hypo-	______________________	**20.** in-	______________________
21. inter-	______________________	**22.** multi-	______________________
23. para-	______________________	**24.** peri-	______________________
25. poly-	______________________	**26.** pre-	______________________
27. re-	______________________	**28.** sub-	______________________
29. super-	______________________	**30.** un-	______________________

Using Prefixes to Build Medical Words

Using a prefix from the following list, build the appropriate medical word.

an-	*hypo-*	*poly-*
bi-	*inter-*	*sub-*
de-	*multi-*	*un-*
hyper-		

1. Pertaining to without jaundice ______________ icteric
2. Nature or quality of excessive activity ______________ active
3. Pertaining to arising from many locations ______________ focal
4. Failure of a system ______________ compensation
5. Pertaining to the microscopic space between cells ______________ cellular
6. The process of having two forks ______________ furcation
7. Pertaining to having more than the normal number of fingers and toes ______________ dactyly
8. Underdevelopment of a tissue, organ, or body ______________ plasia
9. Below sharp ______________ acute
10. Pertaining to not being aware ______________ conscious

Identifying Medical Terms

In the spaces provided, write the medical terms for the following meanings.

1. ______________________ Pertaining to without fever
2. ______________________ Pertaining to outside the eye
3. ______________________ Condition of not being able to sleep
4. ______________________ To stop, inhibit, restrain
5. ______________________ To remove the kernel of
6. ______________________ Space within an artery, vein, intestine, or tube
7. ______________________ Wide open
8. ______________________ To act again
9. ______________________ Any objective evidence of an illness
10. ______________________ Any perceptible change in the function of the body that indicates disease

Study and Review I

Anatomy and Physiology

Write your answers to the following questions.

1. The ______________________ consist of millions of ______________________ working individually and with each other to ______________________ life.

2. The outer covering of the cell is known as the ______________________, which has the capability of allowing some substances to pass into and out of the cell.

3. The common parts of the cell are the ______________________, ______________________, and ______________________.

4. Three functions of the cell's nucleus are ______________________, ______________________, and ______________________.

5. An ______________________ is an unspecialized cell that can turn itself into any type of tissue.

6. List the six functions of epithelial tissue.

   a. ______________________ b. ______________________

   c. ______________________ d. ______________________

   e. ______________________ f. ______________________

7. ______________________ tissue is the most widespread and abundant of the four body tissues.

8. Name the three types of muscle tissue.

   a. ______________________ b. ______________________

   c. ______________________

9. Two properties of nerve tissue are ______________________ and ______________________.

10. Define *organ*. ______________________.

11. Define *body system*. ______________________.

12. Name the organ systems listed in this text.

   a. ______________________ b. ______________________

   c. ______________________ d. ______________________

   e. ______________________ f. ______________________

g. ______________________ h. ______________________

i. ______________________ j. ______________________

k. ______________________

13. Define the following directional terms.

a. superior ______________________ **b.** anterior ______________________

c. posterior ______________________ **d.** cephalic ______________________

e. medial ______________________ **f.** lateral ______________________

g. proximal ______________________ **h.** distal ______________________

14. The ______________________ vertically divides the body. It passes through the midline to form a right and left half.

15. The ______________________ plane is any plane that divides the body into superior and inferior portions.

16. The ______________________ plane is any plane that divides the body at right angles to the plane described in Question 14.

17. List the three distinct cavities that are located in the ventral cavity.

a. ______________________ **b.** ______________________

c. ______________________

18. Name the two distinct cavities located in the dorsal cavity.

a. ______________________ **b.** ______________________

ANATOMY LABELING

Identify the structures shown below by filling in the blanks.

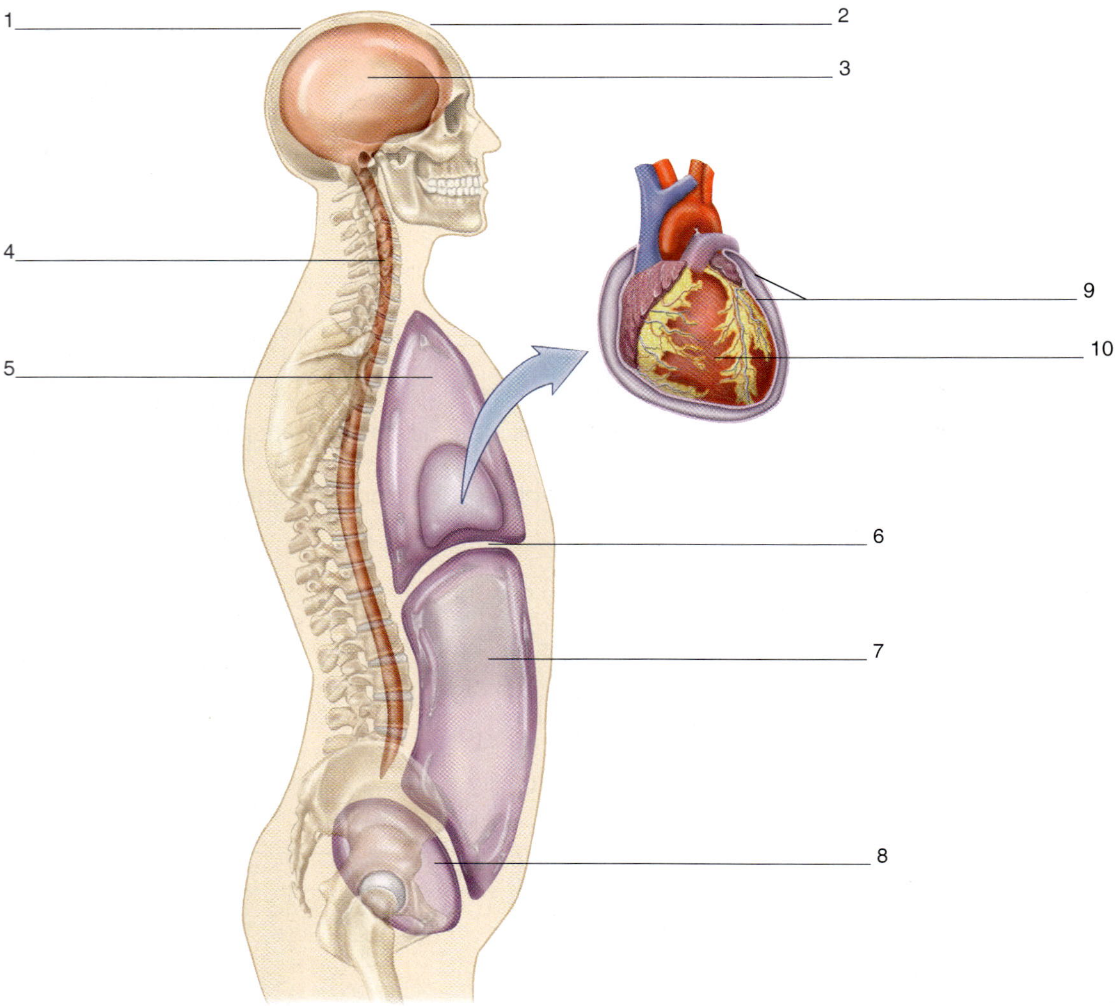

Study and Review II

Word Parts

Prefixes

Give the definitions of the following prefixes.

1. ambi- ______________________
2. ana- ______________________
3. bi- ______________________
4. chromo- ______________________
5. de- ______________________
6. dif- ______________________
7. ecto- ______________________
8. endo- ______________________
9. homeo- ______________________
10. meso- ______________________
11. per- ______________________
12. proto- ______________________
13. uni- ______________________

Combining Forms

Give the definitions of the following combining forms.

1. adip/o ______________________
2. andr/o ______________________
3. anter/o ______________________
4. bi/o ______________________
5. caud/o ______________________
6. cyt/o ______________________
7. dist/o ______________________
8. dors/o ______________________
9. hist/o ______________________
10. hydr/o ______________________
11. infer/o ______________________
12. inguin/o ______________________
13. kary/o ______________________
14. later/o ______________________
15. medi/o ______________________
16. organ/o ______________________
17. path/o ______________________
18. phen/o ______________________
19. physi/o ______________________
20. poster/o ______________________
21. proxim/o ______________________
22. somat/o ______________________
23. ventr/o ______________________
24. viscer/o ______________________

Suffixes

Give the definitions for the following suffixes.

1. -al ______________________
2. -ate ______________________
3. -genesis ______________________
4. -ic ______________________
5. -ion ______________________
6. -logy ______________________
7. -morph ______________________
8. -oid ______________________
9. -ose ______________________
10. -plasm ______________________
11. -some ______________________
12. -stasis ______________________
13. -tomy ______________________
14. -type ______________________

Identifying Medical Terms

In the spaces provided, write the medical terms for the following meanings.

1. ______________________ To resemble man
2. ______________________ Pertaining to two sides
3. ______________________ Study of cells
4. ______________________ Slender physical body form
5. ______________________ Formation of a cell's nucleus
6. ______________________ Pertaining to the stimulation of body growth
7. ______________________ Pertaining to one side

Matching

Select the appropriate lettered meaning for each of the following words.

__________ 1. ambilateral
__________ 2. anatomy
__________ 3. atom
__________ 4. chromosome
__________ 5. cilia
__________ 6. homeostasis
__________ 7. human genome
__________ 8. phenotype
__________ 9. physiology
__________ 10. vertex

a. Hairlike processes that project from epithelial cells
b. Top or highest point
c. Pertaining to both sides
d. Study of the structure of an organism such as a human
e. Smallest, most basic chemical unit of an element
f. Microscopic bodies that carry the genes that determine hereditary characteristics
g. Complete set of genes and chromosomes
h. Physical appearance or type of makeup of an individual
i. State of equilibrium maintained in the body's internal environment
j. Study of the nature of a living organism
k. Study of disease

Study and Review III

Building Medical Terms

Using the following word parts, fill in the blanks to build the correct medical terms.

bi-	inguin	-al
uni-	path/o	-ic
bi/o	physi/o	-logy

Definition	Medical Term
1. Pertaining to both sides	________lateral
2. Study of life	_________logy
3. Farthest from the point of origin	dist__________
4. Pertaining to the groin	___________al
5. Pertaining to the side	later__________
6. Study of disease	_________logy
7. Study of the function of living organisms	_________logy
8. Pertaining to the body as a whole	system_______
9. Pertaining to one side	________lateral
10. Pertaining to body organs enclosed within a cavity	viscer________

Combining Form Challenge

Using the combining forms provided, write the medical term correctly.

adip/o	hist/o	phen/o
andr/o	kary/o	somat/o

1. Pertaining to fatty tissue throughout the body: __________ose
2. To resemble man: ___________oid
3. Study of tissue: ________ logy
4. Formation of a cell's nucleus: ___________genesis
5. Physical appearance or type of makeup of an individual: __________type
6. Pertaining to stimulation of body growth: ________trophic

Select the Right Term

Select the correct answer, and write it on the line provided.

1. Literally means *to cut up* or *to cut apart* is __________.

   physiology **anatomy** **homeostasis** **topical**

2. A surface or part situated toward the front of the body is __________.

   caudal **cranial** **anterior** **medical**

3. A well-proportioned body form is __________.

   endomorph **phenotype** **somatotrophic** **mesomorph**

4. The lower part or foundation of a structure is __________.

   apex **base** **dorsal** **vertex**

5. Nearest the center or point of origin is __________.

   superior **ventral** **topical** **proximal**

6. Pertaining to lying flat, even, level is __________.

   inguinal **horizontal** **medial** **dorsal**

Abbreviations

Place the correct word, phrase, or abbreviation in the space provided.

1. abd ______________________________
2. A&P ______________________________
3. DNA ______________________________
4. body mass index ______________________________
5. gastrointestinal ______________________________
6. H_2O ______________________________
7. LLQ ______________________________
8. oxygen ______________________________
9. over-the-counter (drugs) ______________________________
10. RUQ ______________________________

Practical Application

ICD-10-CM Terminology

Write your answers to the following questions.

1. In ICD-10-CM, morbid (severe) obesity (E66.01) is due to excess ______________.
2. The term ______________ is not recognized as a clinical term for high adiposity obesity.
3. __________ (side of the body affected) is a new coding convention added to the ICD-10-CM.
4. The term ________________ means "substances used for medical treatment."
5. The term ________________ means "taking less of a medication than is prescribed."

Study and Review I

Anatomy and Physiology

Write your answers to the following questions.

1. Name the primary organ of the integumentary system. _______________

2. Name the four accessory structures of the integumentary system.

   a. _______________ b. _______________

   c. _______________ d. _______________

3. State the four main functions of the skin.

   a. _______________ b. _______________

   c. _______________ d. _______________

4. The skin is essentially composed of two layers, the _______________ and the _______________.

5. Name the five strata of the epidermis.

   a. _______________ b. _______________

   c. _______________ d. _______________

   e. _______________

6. _______________ is a protein substance that is the basic structural component of hair and nails.

7. _______________ is a pigment that gives color to the skin.

8. The _______________ is known as the *corium* or *true skin*.

9. Name the two layers of the part of the skin described in question 8.

   a. _______________ b. _______________

10. The crescent-shaped white area of the nail is the _______________.

ANATOMY LABELING

Identify the structures shown below by filling in the blanks.

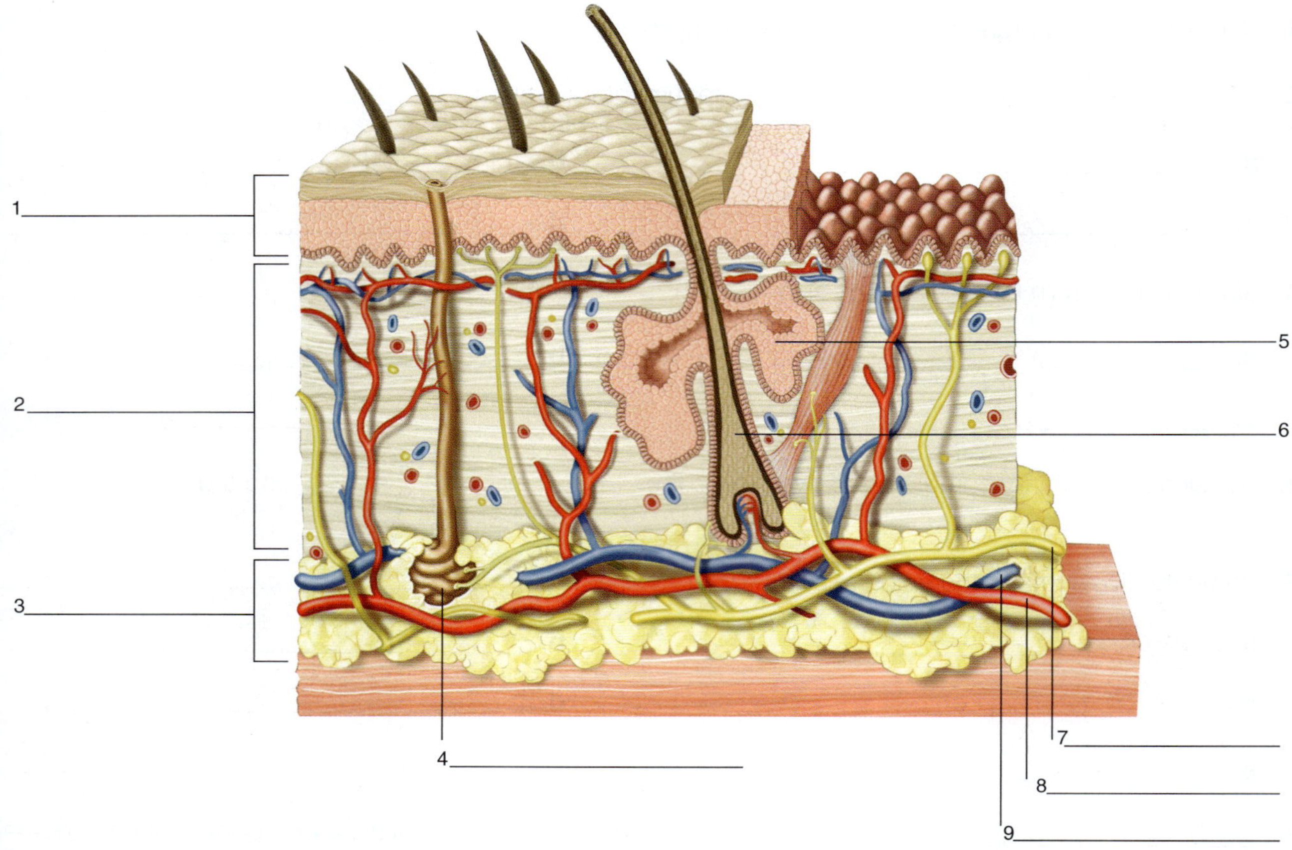

Study and Review II

Word Parts

Prefixes

Give the definitions of the following prefixes.

1. a-, an- ________________
2. auto- ________________
3. ec- ________________
4. de- ________________
5. ex- ________________
6. hyper- ________________
7. hypo- ________________
8. intra- ________________
9. par- ________________
10. sub- ________________

Combining Forms

Give the definitions of the following combining forms.

1. albin/o ________________
2. caus/o ________________
3. cutane/o ________________
4. derm/o ________________
5. erythr/o ________________
6. hidr/o ________________
7. icter/o ________________
8. kel/o ________________
9. kerat/o ________________
10. leuk/o ________________
11. melan/o ________________
12. onych/o ________________
13. pachy/o ________________
14. pedicul/o ________________
15. plak/o ________________
16. prurit/o ________________
17. rhytid/o ________________
18. scler/o ________________
19. seb/o ________________
20. therm/o ________________
21. trich/o ________________
22. vuls/o ________________
23. xanth/o ________________
24. xer/o ________________

Suffixes

Give the definitions of the following suffixes.

1. -al ______________________
2. -algia ______________________
3. -on ______________________
4. -us ______________________
5. -derma ______________________
6. -ary ______________________
7. -esthesia ______________________
8. -graft ______________________
9. -ia ______________________
10. -ic ______________________
11. -ion ______________________
12. -ism ______________________
13. -ist ______________________
14. -itis ______________________
15. -logy ______________________
16. -ectasia ______________________
17. -oid ______________________
18. -oma ______________________
19. -osis ______________________
20. -ous ______________________
21. -plasty ______________________
22. -rrhea ______________________
23. -tome ______________________

Identifying Medical Terms

In the spaces provided, write the medical terms for the following meanings.

1. ______________________ Inflammation of the skin caused by exposure to actinic rays
2. ______________________ Pertaining to the skin
3. ______________________ Inflammation of the skin
4. ______________________ Study of the skin
5. ______________________ Severe itching
6. ______________________ Condition of excessive sweating
7. ______________________ Pertaining to under the skin

8. ______________________ Pertaining to jaundice

9. ______________________ Inflammation of the nail

10. ______________________ Thick skin

11. ______________________ Inability to distinguish between the sensations of heat and cold

12. ______________________ Yellowness of the skin

Matching

Select the appropriate lettered meaning for each of the following words.

__________ **1.** acne

__________ **2.** alopecia

__________ **3.** cicatrix

__________ **4.** comedo

__________ **5.** decubitus

__________ **6.** dehiscence

__________ **7.** exudate

__________ **8.** leukoplakia

__________ **9.** petechiae

__________ **10.** pruritus

a. Small, pinpoint, purplish hemorrhagic spots on the skin

b. Production of pus or serum

c. Severe itching

d. Inflammatory condition of the sebaceous glands and the hair follicles

e. Scar left after the healing of a wound

f. Loss of hair, baldness

g. White spots or patches formed on the mucous membrane of the tongue or cheek

h. Blackhead

i. Separation or bursting open of a surgical wound

j. Bedsore

k. Slough, scab

Medical Case Snapshots

This learning activity provides an opportunity to relate the medical terminology you are learning to a precise patient case presentation. In the spaces provided, write in your answers.

Case 1

A 36-year-old male is concerned about noticeable loss of scalp hair. He states that his cousins on his mother's side have the same thing. The medical term for this condition is ____________ (loss of hair, especially on the scalp). The androgenetic type of this condition (formerly called *male-pattern baldness*) begins in the frontal area and progresses until only a horseshoe-shaped area of hair remains.

Case 2

When the 45-year-old female was asked about her chief complaint she said, "I would like something done to remove the wrinkles from around my eyes and mouth." Dr. Smith, a dermatologist, explained that he could either do a ___________ (surgical procedure to remove fine wrinkles) or he could perform a _______________ (type of plastic surgery).

Case 3

The 84-year-old bedridden patient is diagnosed with a large decubitus ulcer located on her right buttocks. The literal meaning of the word *decubitus* is ____________________.

Study and Review III

Building Medical Terms

Using the following word parts, fill in the blanks to build the correct medical terms.

de-	xanth	-ic
melan	xanth/o	-rrhea
pachy	xer	
onych	-logy	

Definition	Medical Term
1. An area of skin and tissue that becomes broken down	_________ cubitus
2. Study of the skin	dermato________
3. Pertaining to jaundice	icter___________
4. Cancer that develops in the pigment cells of the skin	___________ oma
5. Inflammation of the nail	____________ itis
6. Thick skin	__________derma
7. Excessive flow of oil from the sebaceous glands	sebo ___________
8. Yellowness of the skin	__________ derma
9. Literally means yellow tumor	____________ oma
10. Abnormal dryness of skin	_____________osis

Combining Form Challenge

Using the combining forms provided, write the medical term correctly.

albin/o	cutane/o	erythr/o
caus/o	dermat/o	integument/o

1. Genetic condition in which there is a partial or total absence of pigment in skin, hair, and eyes: __________ ism
2. Intense burning pain associated with trophic skin changes in the hand or foot after trauma to the part: ___________ algia
3. Pertaining to the skin: ________ ous
4. Inflammation of the skin: ___________ itis
5. Abnormal redness of the skin occurring over widespread areas of the body: __________derma
6. Covering; the skin, consisting of the dermis and epidermis: ________ ary

Select the Right Term

Select the correct answer and write it on the line provided.

1. Inflammatory condition of the sebaceous glands and hair follicles is ____________.

actinic dermatitis **bite** **boil** **acne**

2. The absence or loss of hair, especially of the head, is _________.

acrochordon **alopecia** **anhidrosis** **avulsion**

3. Scar left after the healing of a wound is _______________.

boil **burn** **corn** **cicatrix**

4. Slough, scab is _______________.

eschar **exudate** **folliculitis** **gangrene**

5. A flat, brownish spot on the skin; freckle is ______________.

keloid **lupus** **lentigo** **mole**

6. Any rose-colored rash marked by maculae or red spots on the skin is _______.

rosacea **roseola** **rubella** **robeola**

Diagnostic and Laboratory Tests

Select the best answer to each multiple-choice question. Circle the letter of your choice.

1. An intradermal test performed using a sterile, disposable, multiple-puncture lancet is called a ______________

a. sweat test.
b. Mantoux test.
c. tine test.
d. Tzanck test.

2. A test done on wound exudate to determine the presence of microorganisms is called a _________________

a. sweat test.
b. biopsy.
c. Tzanck test.
d. wound culture.

3. A microscopic examination of a small piece of tissue that has been surgically scraped from a pustule is called a ________________________

a. Tzanck test.
b. sweat test.
c. biopsy.
d. wound culture.

4. Tests performed to identify the presence of the *Tubercle bacilli* include the ___________________________

a. tine, Heaf, and sweat tests.
b. tine, Heaf, and Mantoux tests.
c. tine, Tzanck, and Mantoux tests.
d. tine, Mantoux, and sweat tests.

5. The ________________________ test is used to determine the level of chloride concentration on the skin.

a. sweat
b. Tzanck
c. tine
d. Mantoux

Abbreviations

Place the correct word, phrase, or abbreviation in the space provided.

1. basal cell carcinoma ______________________________
2. Bx ______________________________
3. decub ______________________________
4. ID ______________________________
5. SCC ______________________________
6. PPD ______________________________
7. skin graft ______________________________
8. staph ______________________________
9. strep ______________________________
10. topical immunomodulators ______________________________

Practical Application

Medical Record Analysis

This exercise contains information, abbreviations, and medical terminology from an actual medical record or case study that has been adapted for this text. The names and any personal information have been created by the author. Read and study each form or case study and then answer the questions that follow. You may refer to Appendix III, *Abbreviations and Symbols*.

SOUTH SIDE PATHOLOGY, PC

Task Edit View Time Scale Options Help Date: 17 May 2017

315 West Eighth Street • Rome, GA 30165
Phone: 123-456-7890
Frank Jones Smith, MD, Laboratory Director

Surgical Pathology Report

Patient: Frances Marie Melton
DOB: 1/31/45
Gender: Female
Age: 72
Signed: Scott Parker, MD
Northside Dermatology
103 John Maddox Drive
Rome, GA 30165

Case Number: 104589
Collected: 02/11/2017
Received: 02/12/2017

Clinical Information:

1. Hemorrhagic papule Dx: BCC
2. Translucent papule with telangiectasia Dx: BCC

Diagnosis:
1. Skin of left nasal dorsum, shave biopsy—actinic keratosis.
2. Skin of right mid back, shave biopsy—basal cell carcinoma.

Gross Description:
1. Two containers, the first labeled "left nasal dorsum," have within a brown and white 4 × 5 mm superficial skin shave. With margins inked, this is bisected and entirely submitted.
2. The second, labeled "right mid back," has within a 0.5 × 0.7 cm superficial skin shave. With margins inked, this is trisected and entirely submitted.

Microscopic Description:

1. Sections show keratinocyte atypical involving the lower layers of the epidermis as well as solar elastosis (breakdown of elastic tissue due to apparent excessive sun exposure) and parakeratosis (incomplete keratinization due to apparent excessive sun exposure). The actinic keratosis has proliferative features.
2. Sections show a mixed superficial and micronodular form of basal cell carcinoma featuring focal pigmentation. The lesion extends to the base of the shave.

Frank Jones Smith, MD
Pathologist
(Case signed 02/14/2017)

Medical Record Questions

Place the correct answer in the space provided.

1. What is the abbreviation for diagnosis? ____________________
2. What does the abbreviation BCC mean? ____________________
3. Define papule. ____________________
4. What is the medical term that means dilatation of small blood vessels that may appear as a birthmark? ____________________
5. What is the medical term that means breakdown of elastic tissue due to apparent excessive sun exposure? ____________________

Study and Review I

Anatomy and Physiology

Write your answers to the following questions.

1. The skeletal system is composed of ______________ bones.

2. Name the two main divisions of the skeletal system.

   a. ______________ b. ______________

3. Name five classifications of bone and give an example of each.

   a. ______________ Example: ______________

   b. ______________ Example: ______________

   c. ______________ Example: ______________

   d. ______________ Example: ______________

   e. ______________ Example: ______________

4. State the six main functions of bones.

   a. ______________ b. ______________

   c. ______________ d. ______________

   e. ______________ f. ______________

5. Define the following features of a long bone.

   a. Epiphysis ______________

   b. Diaphysis ______________

   c. Periosteum ______________

   d. Compact bone ______________

   e. Medullary canal ______________

   f. Endosteum ______________

   g. Cancellous or spongy bone ______________

6. Match the term in the left column with its definition from the right. Place the correct letter from the right column in the space provided in the left column.

______ 1. meatus	a. Air cavity within certain bones
______ 2. head	b. Shallow depression in or on a bone
______ 3. tuberosity	c. Pointed, sharp, slender process
______ 4. process	d. Large, rounded process
______ 5. condyle	e. Groove, furrow, depression, or fissure
______ 6. tubercle	f. Tubelike passage or canal
______ 7. crest	g. Opening in the bone for blood vessels, ligaments, and nerves
______ 8. trochanter	h. Rounded projection that enters into the formation of a joint, articulation
______ 9. sinus	i. Ridge on a bone
______ 10. fissure	j. Small, rounded process
______ 11. fossa	k. Rounded end of a bone
______ 12. spine	l. Slitlike opening between two bones
______ 13. foramen	m. Enlargement or protrusion of a bone
______ 14. sulcus	n. Either of the two bony projections below the neck of the femur

7. Name the three classifications of joints.

a. ______________________ b. ______________________

c. ______________________

8. ______________________ is moving a body part away from the middle.

9. Adduction is ____.

10. ______________________ is moving a body part in a circular motion.

11. Dorsiflexion is ____.

12. ______________________ is turning outward.

13. Extension is ____.

14. ______________________ is bending a limb.

15. Inversion is ______________________________.

16. ______________________ is lying face downward.

17. Protraction is ______________________________.

18. ______________________ is moving a body part backward.

19. Rotation is ______________________________.

20. ______________________ is lying face upward.

ANATOMY LABELING

Identify the structures shown below by filling in the blanks.

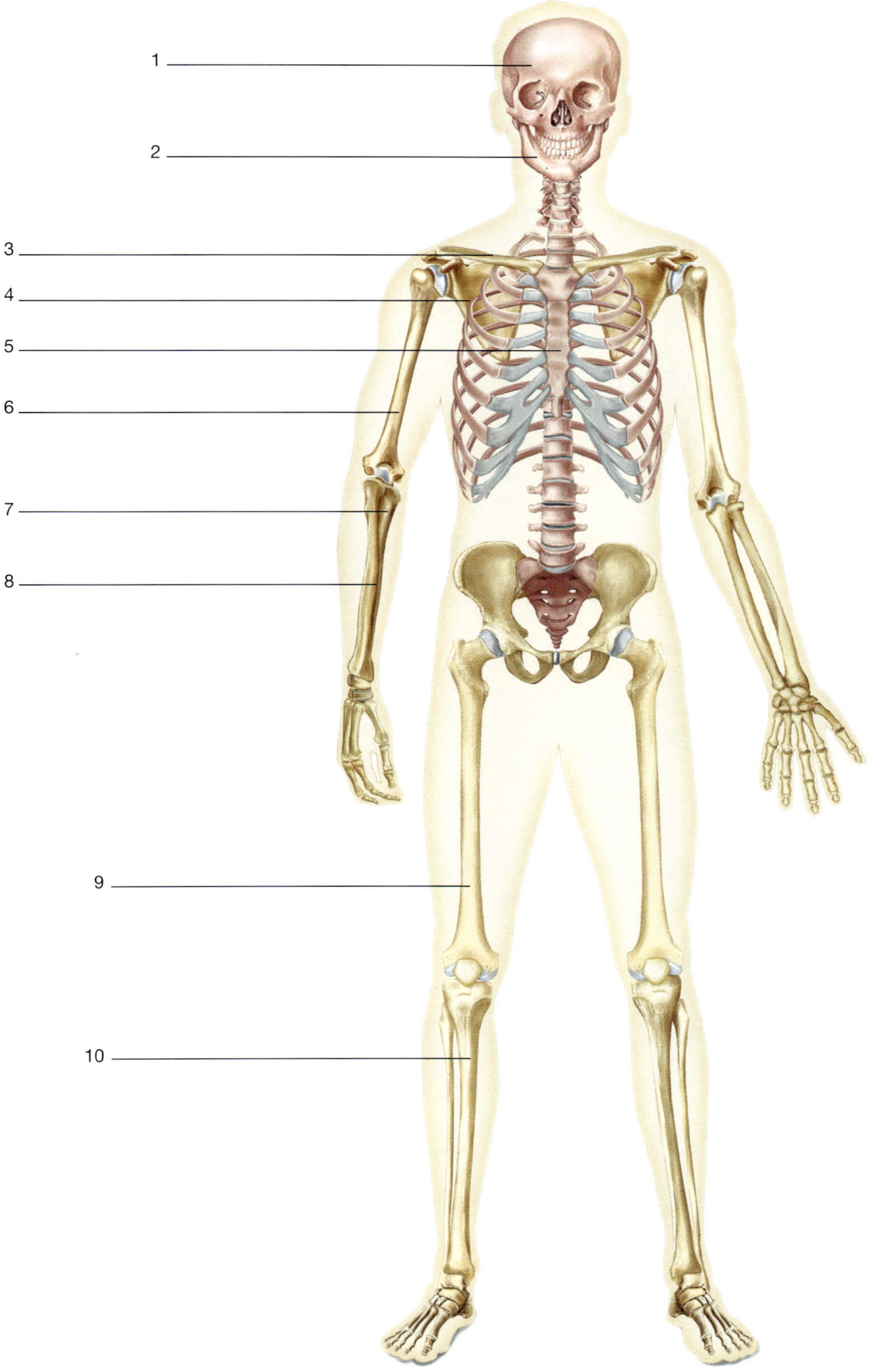

Study and Review II

Word Parts

Prefixes

Give the definitions of the following prefixes.

1. a- ____________________
2. dis- ____________________
3. hydr- ____________________
4. inter- ____________________
5. meta- ____________________
6. peri- ____________________
7. poly- ____________________
8. sub- ____________________
9. sym- ____________________
10. re- ____________________

Combining Forms

Give the definitions of the following combining forms.

1. acr/o ____________________
2. ankyl/o ____________________
3. arthr/o ____________________
4. burs/o ____________________
5. calcan/e ____________________
6. carp/o ____________________
7. chondr/o ____________________
8. coccyg/o ____________________
9. cost/o ____________________
10. crani/o ____________________
11. dactyl/o ____________________
12. isch/i ____________________
13. kyph/o ____________________
14. lord/o ____________________
15. lumb/o ____________________
16. oste/o ____________________
17. patell/o ____________________
18. ped/o ____________________
19. sacr/o ____________________
20. scoli/o ____________________
21. spin/o ____________________
22. stern/o ____________________
23. uln/o ____________________
24. xiph/o ____________________

Suffixes

Give the definitions of the following suffixes.

1. -ac ______________________
2. -al ______________________
3. -algia ______________________
4. -ar ______________________
5. -ary ______________________
6. -blast ______________________
7. -centesis ______________________
8. -age ______________________
9. -ion ______________________
10. -dynia ______________________
11. -ectomy ______________________
12. -edema ______________________
13. -gen ______________________
14. -genesis ______________________
15. -gram ______________________
16. -graph ______________________
17. -ic ______________________
18. -itis ______________________
19. -ive ______________________
20. -scope ______________________
21. -malacia ______________________
22. -us ______________________
23. -oid ______________________
24. -oma ______________________
25. -osis ______________________
26. -penia ______________________
27. -physis ______________________
28. -plasia ______________________
29. -plasty ______________________
30. -poiesis ______________________
31. -tome ______________________
32. -tomy ______________________
33. -um ______________________

Identifying Medical Terms

In the spaces provided, write the medical terms for the following meanings.

1. ______________________ Inflammation of the joints of the hands or feet
2. ______________________ Abnormal condition of stiffening of a joint
3. ______________________ Inflammation of a joint
4. ______________________ Pertaining to the heel bone
5. ______________________ Pertaining to cartilage
6. ______________________ Pain in the coccyx

7. ______________________ Pertaining to the rib cartilage

8. ______________________ Surgical excision of a portion of the skull

9. ______________________ Pertaining to the finger or toe

10. ______________________ Surgical instrument used for cutting bone

11. ______________________ Pertaining to the space between two ribs

12. ______________________ Pain in the hip

13. ______________________ Pertaining to the loins

14. ______________________ Tumor of the bone marrow

15. ______________________ Inflammation of the bone and joint

16. ______________________ Inflammation of the bone marrow

17. ______________________ Deficiency of bone tissue

18. ______________________ Pertaining to the foot

19. ______________________ Literally means resembling a sword

Matching

Select the appropriate lettered meaning for each of the following words.

________ **1.** arthroscope

________ **2.** carpal tunnel syndrome

________ **3.** fixation

________ **4.** gout

________ **5.** hammertoe

________ **6.** kyphosis

________ **7.** metacarpal

________ **8.** rickets

________ **9.** tennis elbow

________ **10.** ulnar

a. Abnormal condition that can occur in children and is caused by a lack of vitamin D

b. An acquired flexion deformity of the interphalangeal joint

c. Hereditary metabolic disease that is a form of acute arthritis

d. Chronic condition characterized by elbow pain that is caused by excessive pronation and supination activities of the forearm

e. Making rigid, immobilizing

f. Pertaining to the ulna (long bone of the forearm between the wrist and elbow), or to the nerve or artery named for it

g. Pertaining to the bones of the hand

h. In this condition, the normal thoracic curvature becomes exaggerated, producing a "humpback" appearance

i. Surgical instrument used to examine the interior of a joint

j. Abnormal condition caused by compression of the median nerve by the carpal ligament

k. Pertaining to the knee

Medical Case Snapshots

This learning activity provides an opportunity to relate the medical terminology you are learning to a precise patient case presentation. In the spaces provided, write in your answers.

Case 1

A 66-year-old female is scheduled for a dual-energy x-ray absorptiometry (DXA) scan, to measure her bone mineral density. She is diagnosed with osteoarthritis. The results of her test show ______________ (deficiency of bone tissue) and ____________ (which is characterized by a decrease in bone density).

Case 2

A 4-year-old female is seen by an orthopedic specialist. Upon physical examination an abnormal lateral curvature of the spine, known as ____________, was noted. The characteristic signs of this condition include _____________ of the trunk, uneven shoulders and hips, a one-sided rib hump, and a prominent __________.

Case 3

Upon a return visit to her physician, Ms. Anita Sinclair presented with symptoms of inflammation of the joints, stiffness, pain, and swelling, especially of both hands. This condition is referred to as ______________ _______________ (RA). The multisystem effects of this condition are varied. See Figure 6.18.

Study and Review III

Building Medical Terms

Using the following word parts, fill in the blanks to build the correct medical terms.

dactyl	oste/o	scoli
meta-	patell	-al
-dynia	-poiesis	-osis
-oid		

Definition	Medical Term
1. Pain in the coccyx (tailbone)	coccygo______
2. Pertaining to the finger or toe	___________ic
3. An abnormal anterior curvature of the lumbar spine	lord__________
4. Pertaining to the bones of the hand	________carpals
5. Formation of bone marrow	myelo________
6. Softening of bone	_______malacia
7. Pertaining to the kneecap	___________ar
8. Pertaining to the bones of the fingers and the toes	phalange______
9. An abnormal lateral curvature of the spine	__________osis
10. Literally means resembling a sword	xiph__________

Combining Form Challenge

Using the combining forms provided, write the medical term correctly.

arthr/o	carp/o	cost/o
burs/o	chondr/o	dactyl/o

1. Surgical procedure used to repair a joint: ____________plasty

2. Inflammation of a bursa: ___________itis

3. Pertaining to the wrist: ___________al

4. Pertaining to cartilage: __________al

5. Pertaining to the rib cartilage: __________al

6. Medical term for fingerprint: _________gram

Select the Right Term

Select the correct answer, and write it on the line provided.

1. Abnormal condition of stiffening of a joint is ______________.

   acroarthritis **acromion** **ankylosis** **arthrocentesis**

2. Surgical excision of a portion of the skull is ________.

   craniectomy **craniotomy** **cranectomy** **cranotomy**

3. Pain in the hip is ______________.

   ischial **ischialgia** **ischalgia** **ischial**

4. Pertaining to the lower jaw is ______________.

   maxillary **meniscus** **mandiblar** **mandibular**

5. Malignant tumor of the bone; cancer growing from cells of "fleshy" connective tissue is ______________.

   osteocarcioma **osteosarcoma** **osteogenesis** **myeloma**

6. Surgery performed to permanently connect two or more vertebrae in the spine is ______________.

   myelitis **acroarthritis** **spondylodesis** **vertebral**

Diagnostic and Laboratory Tests

Select the best answer to each multiple-choice question. Circle the letter of your choice.

1. __________________ is a diagnostic examination of a joint in which air and then a radiopaque contrast medium are injected into the joint space, x-rays are taken, and internal injuries of the meniscus, cartilage, and ligaments may be seen, if present.

   a. Arthroscopy
   b. Goniometry
   c. Arthrography
   d. Thermography

2. The process of recording heat patterns of the body's surface is ___________.

   a. arthrography
   b. arthroscopy
   c. goniometry
   d. thermography

3. __________________ is increased in gout, arthritis, multiple myeloma, and rheumatism.

   a. Calcium
   b. Phosphorus
   c. Uric acid
   d. Alkaline phosphatase

4. The __________________ level of the blood can be increased in osteoporosis and fracture healing.

   a. antinuclear antibodies
   b. phosphorus
   c. uric acid
   d. alkaline phosphatase

5. __________________ is/are present in a variety of immunological diseases.

   a. Alkaline phosphatase
   b. Antinuclear antibodies
   c. C-reactive protein
   d. Uric acid

Abbreviations

Place the correct word, phrase, or abbreviation in the space provided.

1. antinuclear antibodies ______________________
2. fracture ______________________
3. LLC ______________________
4. OA ______________________
5. phosphorus ______________________
6. RA ______________________
7. range of motion ______________________
8. T1 ______________________
9. TNF ______________________
10. traction ______________________

Practical Application

Medical Record Analysis

This exercise contains information, abbreviations, and medical terminology from an actual medical record or case study that has been adapted for this text. The names and any personal information have been created by the author. Read and study each form or case study and then answer the questions that follow. You may refer to Appendix III, *Abbreviations and Symbols*.

CLEAR SHOT IMAGING SERVICES

Task Edit View Time Scale Options Help Date: 17 May 2017

Phone (123) 456–7890

NAME: BELL, CRYSTAL JANE ORD: 07DX00145

DATE OF BIRTH: 5/26/51

CLINICAL DATA: v49.81 POST MENO

REQUESTING PHYSICIAN: Kyle Preston, MD

EXAM CODE: XRDXA/76075 ORDER DATE: 03/19/2017

LOCATION: SHORTER MEDICAL

EXAM: XR DXA, BONE DENSITY SCAN, 03/19/2017

BONE DENSITOMETRY, 3/19/2017

Routine bone densitometry of the lumbar spine and both hips was performed. The results of the examination expressed as standard deviations (SDs) from the mean bone mineral density (BMD) are as follows:

Spine (L1–L4) T-score	0.6	Z-score	1.7
Femoral neck T-score	–2.3	Z-score	–0.8

Impression:

There is a discrepancy between the lumbar spine and hips due to what I believe is spondylosis. The hips are of a more accurate reading and is consistent with osteopenia. Follow-up in 18–24 months is recommended.

DICTATED: Lions, Daniel

TECHNOLOGIST: 303768

transcribed: rs 03/19/2017

24599

VERIFIED: Daniel Lions, MD

Medical Record Questions

Place the correct answer in the space provided.

1. What is the meaning of DXA? ______________________________
2. What does the abbreviation BMD mean? ______________________________
3. What does the abbreviation L1 mean? ______________________________
4. What is the medical term that means deficiency of bone tissue? ______________________________
5. What is the exam code for this bone density scan? ______________________________

Study and Review I

Anatomy and Physiology

Write your answers to the following questions.

1. The muscular system is made up of three types of muscle tissue. Name the three types.

   a. ______________________ **b.** ______________________

   c. ______________________

2. Muscles make up approximately ______________ percent of a person's body weight.

3. Name the two essential ingredients that are needed for a muscle to perform properly.

   a. ______________________ **b.** ______________________

4. Name the two points of attachment for a skeletal muscle.

   a. ______________________ **b.** ______________________

5. Skeletal muscle is also known as ______________________ or ______________________.

6. A wide, thin, sheetlike tendon is known as an ______________________.

7. Name the three distinguishable parts of a muscle.

   a. ______________________ **b.** ______________________

   c. ______________________

8. Define the following:

a. Antagonist ______________________________

b. Prime mover ______________________________

c. Synergist ______________________________

9. Smooth muscle is also called ______________, ______________, or ______________.

10. Smooth muscles are found in the internal organs. Name five examples of these locations.

a. ______________ **b.** ______________

c. ______________ **d.** ______________

e. ______________

11. ______________ is the muscle of the heart.

12. Name the three primary functions of the muscular system.

a. ______________ **b.** ______________

c. ______________

ANATOMY LABELING

Identify the structures shown below by filling in the blanks.

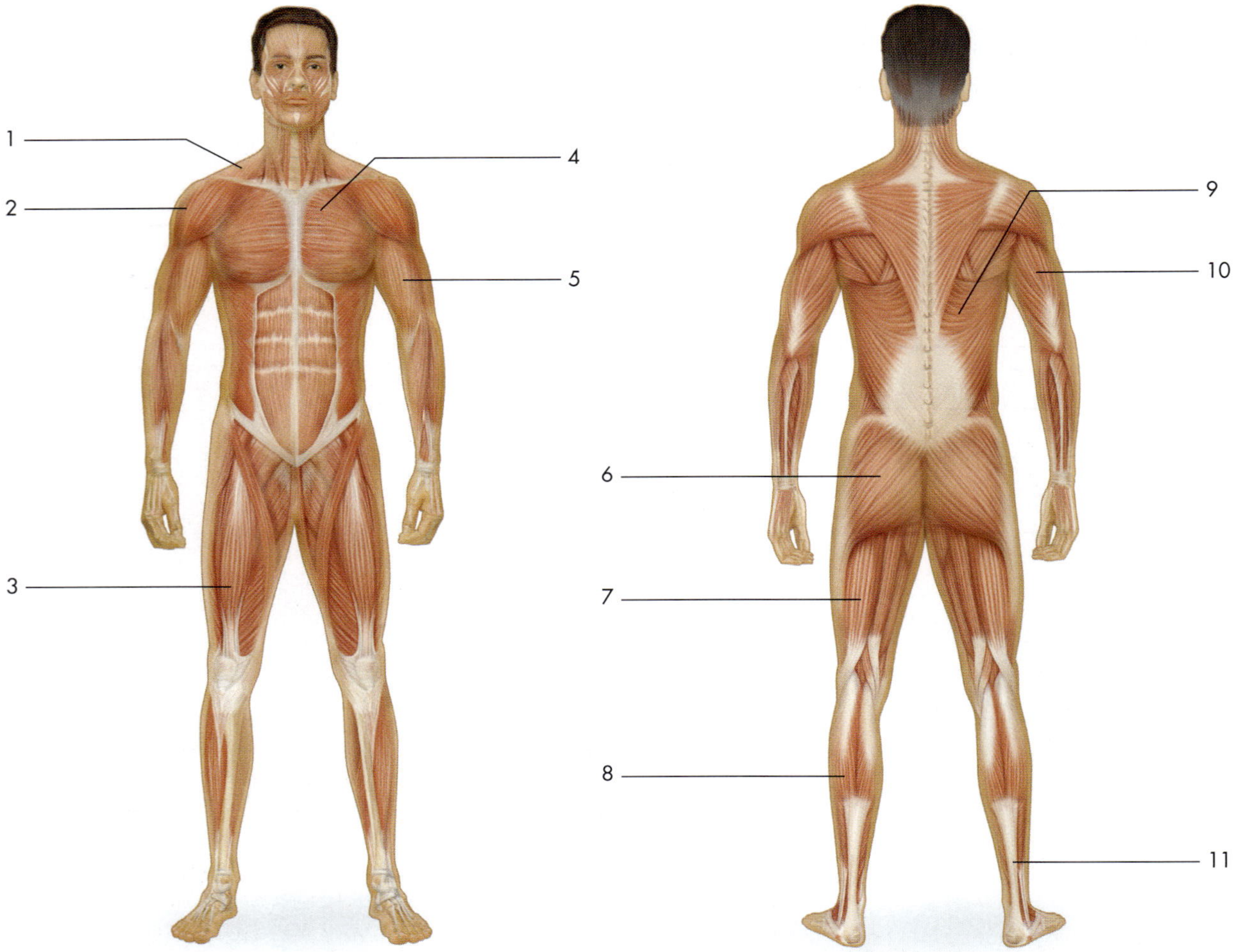

Study and Review II

Word Parts

Prefixes

Give the definitions of the following prefixes.

1. a- ______________________
2. ab- ______________________
3. ad- ______________________
4. ant- ______________________
5. bi- ______________________
6. brady- ______________________
7. con- ______________________
8. dia- ______________________
9. dys- ______________________
10. in- ______________________
11. intra- ______________________
12. hydro- ______________________
13. quadri- ______________________
14. syn- ______________________
15. tri- ______________________

Combining Forms

Give the definitions of the following combining forms.

1. agon/o ______________________
2. amputat/o ______________________
3. brach/i ______________________
4. cleid/o ______________________
5. clon/o ______________________
6. duct/o ______________________
7. fasci/o ______________________
8. fibr/o ______________________
9. is/o ______________________
10. metr/o ______________________
11. muscul/o ______________________
12. my/o ______________________
13. neur/o ______________________
14. path/o ______________________
15. prosth/e ______________________
16. rhabd/o ______________________
17. rotat/o ______________________
18. sarc/o ______________________
19. synov/o ______________________
20. ten/o ______________________
21. ton/o ______________________
22. tors/o ______________________
23. troph/o ______________________
24. volunt/o ______________________

Suffixes

Give the definitions of the following suffixes.

1.	-algia	____________________	**2.**	-ar	____________________
3.	-ary	____________________	**4.**	-asthenia	____________________
5.	-blast	____________________	**6.**	-ceps	____________________
7.	-desis	____________________	**8.**	-dynia	____________________
9.	-in	____________________	**10.**	-therapy	____________________
11.	-graph	____________________	**12.**	-ia	____________________
13.	-ic	____________________	**14.**	-ion	____________________
15.	-ist	____________________	**16.**	-itis	____________________
17.	-ity	____________________	**18.**	-kinesia	____________________
19.	-kinesis	____________________	**20.**	-logy	____________________
21.	-ure	____________________	**22.**	-malacia	____________________
23.	-oid	____________________	**24.**	-oma	____________________
25.	-or	____________________	**26.**	-osis	____________________
27.	-paresis	____________________	**28.**	-pathy	____________________
29.	-phragm	____________________	**30.**	-plasty	____________________
31.	-plegia	____________________	**32.**	-rrhaphy	____________________
33.	-y	____________________	**34.**	-spasm	____________________
35.	-taxia	____________________	**36.**	-tome	____________________
37.	-tomy	____________________	**38.**	-trophy	____________________
39.	-sis	____________________	**40.**	-ism	____________________

Identifying Medical Terms

In the spaces provided, write the medical terms for the following meanings.

1. ____________________ Pertaining to a lack of normal tone or tension

2. ____________________ Slowness of motion or movement

3. ____________________ Medical term for cramp of a finger or toe

4. ______________________ Any condition of abnormal development caused by defective nourishment, often noted by the degeneration of muscles

5. ______________________ Pertaining to within a muscle, such as an IM injection

6. ______________________ Muscle that raises or elevates a part

7. ______________________ Chronic autoimmune neuromuscular disease characterized by varying degrees of weakness of the skeletal (voluntary) muscles of the body

8. ______________________ Weakness or slight paralysis of a muscle

9. ______________________ Surgical repair of a muscle

10. ______________________ Malignant tumor derived from muscle tissue

11. ______________________ Surgical incision into a muscle

12. ______________________ Paralysis affecting many muscles

13. ______________________ Surgical binding of a tendon

14. ______________________ Pertaining to certain muscles that work together

15. ______________________ Muscle having three heads with a single insertion

Matching

Select the appropriate lettered meaning for each of the following words.

______ **1.** dermatomyositis
______ **2.** fibromyalgia
______ **3.** muscular dystrophy
______ **4.** flaccid
______ **5.** prosthesis
______ **6.** rotator cuff
______ **7.** strain
______ **8.** tenodynia
______ **9.** torsion
______ **10.** voluntary

a. Group of muscles and their tendons that act to stabilize the shoulder
b. Process of being twisted
c. Pain in a tendon
d. Chronic immunological disease with systemic pathology
e. Lacking muscle tone; *weak*, *soft*, and *flabby*
f. Under the control of one's will
g. Refers to a group of genetic diseases characterized by progressive weakness and degeneration of the skeletal or voluntary muscles that control movement
h. Excessive, forcible stretching of a muscle or the musculotendinous unit
i. A chronic widespread musculoskeletal pain and fatigue disorder
j. Artificial device used to replace an organ or a body part, such as a hand, arm, leg, or hip
k. Pain in a joint

Medical Case Snapshots

This learning activity provides an opportunity to relate the medical terminology you are learning to a precise patient case presentation. In the spaces provided, write in your answers.

Case 1

The 30-year-old female states, "I feel so tired all the time. I can't sleep at night and my muscles ache." The diagnosis is abbreviated FMS. The American College of Rheumatology classifies a patient with ____________ (FMS) if at least 11 of 18 trigger points are painful under pressure. This patient had 12 trigger points including tiredness or fatigue, and muscle pain or ____________.

Case 2

The mother of a 3-year-old boy states that her son is beginning to appear "clumsy" with increasing episodes of falling. He has trouble getting back up to his feet and has to use his upper body to arise. The physician suspects early onset of ____________ ____________, a term for a group of genetic diseases characterized by progressive weakness and degeneration of the skeletal muscles. The ____________ maneuver is the use of the upper extremity muscles to raise oneself to a standing position. (See Figure 7.12.)

Case 3

The instructor thought it would be a fun and educational experience to ask her students to stand and demonstrate the standard anatomic position. The student should stand with his or her ____________ ____________, head facing ____________, arms by the sides with ____________ to the front. (See Table 7.3.)

Study and Review III

Building Medical Terms

Using the following word parts, fill in the blanks to build the correct medical terms.

a-	ten/o	-graph
bi-	-ion	-lemma
poly-	-ary	
rhabd/o	-or	

Definition	Medical Term
1. Surgical removal of a limb, part, or other appendage	amputat______
2. Lack of muscular coordination	_________taxia
3. Muscle with two points of origin	_________ceps
4. Muscle that raises or elevates a part	levat_________
5. Instrument used to record muscular contractions	myo_________
6. Paralysis affecting many muscles	_________plegia
7. Tumor of striated muscle tissue	_______myoma
8. Plasma membrane surrounding each striated muscle fiber	sarco_________
9. Pain in a tendon	_________dynia
10. Under the control of one's will	volunt________

Combining Form Challenge

Using the combining forms provided, write the medical term correctly.

brach/i	fasci/o	my/o
dactyl/o	is/o	sarc/o

1. Pain in the arm: __________algia

2. Medical term for cramp of a finger or toe: ______________spasm

3. Inflammation of a fascia: ______________itis

4. Literally means pertaining to having equal measure: _____________metric

5. Weakness or slight paralysis of a muscle: ______________paresis

6. Plasma membrane surrounding each striated muscle fiber: _____________lemma

Select the Right Term

Select the correct answer, and write it on the line provided.

1. Muscle that counteracts the action of another muscle is ______________.

   adductor **aponeurosis** **antagonist** **atrophy**

2. Pertains to alternate contraction and relaxation of muscles is ____________.

   bradykinesia **clonic** **contracture** **dystonia**

3. Lacking muscle tone; weak, soft, and flabby is _____________.

   isotonic **myokinesis** **flaccid** **relaxation**

4. Surgical repair of a muscle is ______________.

   myopathy **myoplasty** **myorrhaphy** **myotome**

5. Pertaining to certain muscles that work together is _____________.

   synergetic **synovitis** **adductor** **tetany**

6. Process of being twisted is ______________.

   triceps **torticollis** **tonic** **tenodesis**

Diagnostic and Laboratory Tests

Select the best answer to each multiple-choice question. Circle the letter of your choice.

1. Diagnostic test to help diagnose Duchenne muscular dystrophy before symptoms appear.
   a. creatine kinase
   b. aldolase blood test
   c. calcium blood test
   d. muscle biopsy
2. Test to measure electrical activity across muscle membranes by means of electrodes that are attached to a needle that is inserted into the muscle.
   a. muscle biopsy
   b. lactic dehydrogenase
   c. creatine kinase
   d. electromyography
3. Blood test to determine the level of _________ enzyme, which is increased in skeletal muscle damage and muscular dystrophy, is:
   a. lactic dehydrogenase
   b. aspartate aminotransferase
   c. aldolase
   d. creatine kinase
4. Blood test to determine the level of ____________ enzyme, which is increased in skeletal muscle damage is:
   a. lactic dehydrogenase
   b. aldolase
   c. alanine aminotransferase
   d. creatine kinase
5. A/an ______________________________ is the surgical removal of a small piece of muscle tissue for examination.
   a. muscle biopsy
   b. electromyography
   c. bone biopsy
   d. electrocardiography

Abbreviations

Place the correct word, phrase, or abbreviation in the space provided.

1. AE ______
2. AST ______
3. calcium ______
4. electromyography ______
5. FROM ______
6. MS ______
7. range of motion ______
8. MG ______
9. MD ______
10. FMS ______

Practical Application

Medical Record Analysis

This exercise contains information, abbreviations, and medical terminology from an actual medical record or case study that has been adapted for this text. The names and any personal information have been created by the author. Read and study each form or case study and then answer the questions that follow. You may refer to Appendix III, *Abbreviations and Symbols*.

CASE STUDY: DUCHENNE MUSCULAR DYSTROPHY

Task   Edit   View   Time Scale   Options   Help   Date: 17 May 2017

A 3-year-old male child was seen by a physician; the following is a synopsis of the visit.

Present History: The mother states that she noticed that her son has been falling a lot and seems to be very clumsy. She says that he has a waddling gait, is very slow in running and climbing, and walks on his toes. She is most concerned as she is at risk for carrying the gene that causes muscular dystrophy (MD).

Signs and Symptoms: A waddling gait, very slow in running and climbing, walks on his toes, frequent falling, clumsy.

Diagnosis: Duchenne muscular dystrophy. The diagnosis was determined by the characteristic symptoms, family history, a muscle biopsy, an electromyography (EMG), and an elevated serum creatine kinase (CK) level.

Treatment: Physical therapy, deep breathing exercises to help delay muscular weakness, supportive measures such as splints and braces to help minimize deformities and to preserve mobility. Counseling and referral services are essential. For more information and resources, the family may visit the website of the Muscular Dystrophy Association at *www.mda.org*.

Case Study Questions

Place the correct answer in the space provided.

1. Signs and symptoms of Duchenne muscular dystrophy include a ______________________ gait, frequent falls, clumsiness, slowness in running and climbing, and walking on toes.
2. The diagnosis was determined by the characteristic symptoms, family history, a muscle biopsy, an ______________________, and an elevated serum creatine kinase level.
3. As part of the treatment for Duchenne muscular dystrophy, the use of splints and braces help to (a) ______________________ and (b) ______________________.
4. Define electromyography. ______________________
5. Define muscle biopsy. ______________________

Study and Review I

Anatomy and Physiology

Write your answers to the following questions.

1. Name the primary organs commonly associated with digestion.

   a. ______________________ b. ______________________

   c. ______________________ d. ______________________

   e. ______________________ f. ______________________

2. Name four accessory organs of digestion.

   a. ______________________ b. ______________________

   c. ______________________ d. ______________________

3. State the three main functions of the digestive system.

   a. ______________________ b. ______________________

   c. ______________________

4. Define bolus. ______________________

5. Define peristalsis. ______________________

6. ______________________ and ______________________ convert the food into a semiliquid state.

7. The ______________________ is the first portion of the small intestine.

8. Semiliquid food is called ______________________.

9. The ______________________ transports nutrients to body cells.

10. The large intestine can be divided into four distinct sections called the ______________________, the ______________________, the ______________________, and the ______________________.

11. The ______________________ is the largest glandular organ in the body.

12. State the function of the gallbladder. ______________________

13. Name an important function of the pancreas. ______________________

14. State three functions of the liver.

a. ______________________________ **b.** ______________________________

c. ______________________________

15. Where does digestion and absorption chiefly take place? ______________________________

16. The salivary glands located in and about the mouth are called the ________________________, the ________________________, and the ________________________.

17. Name the two hormones secreted into the bloodstream by the pancreas. ________________________

ANATOMY LABELING

Identify the structures shown below by filling in the blanks.

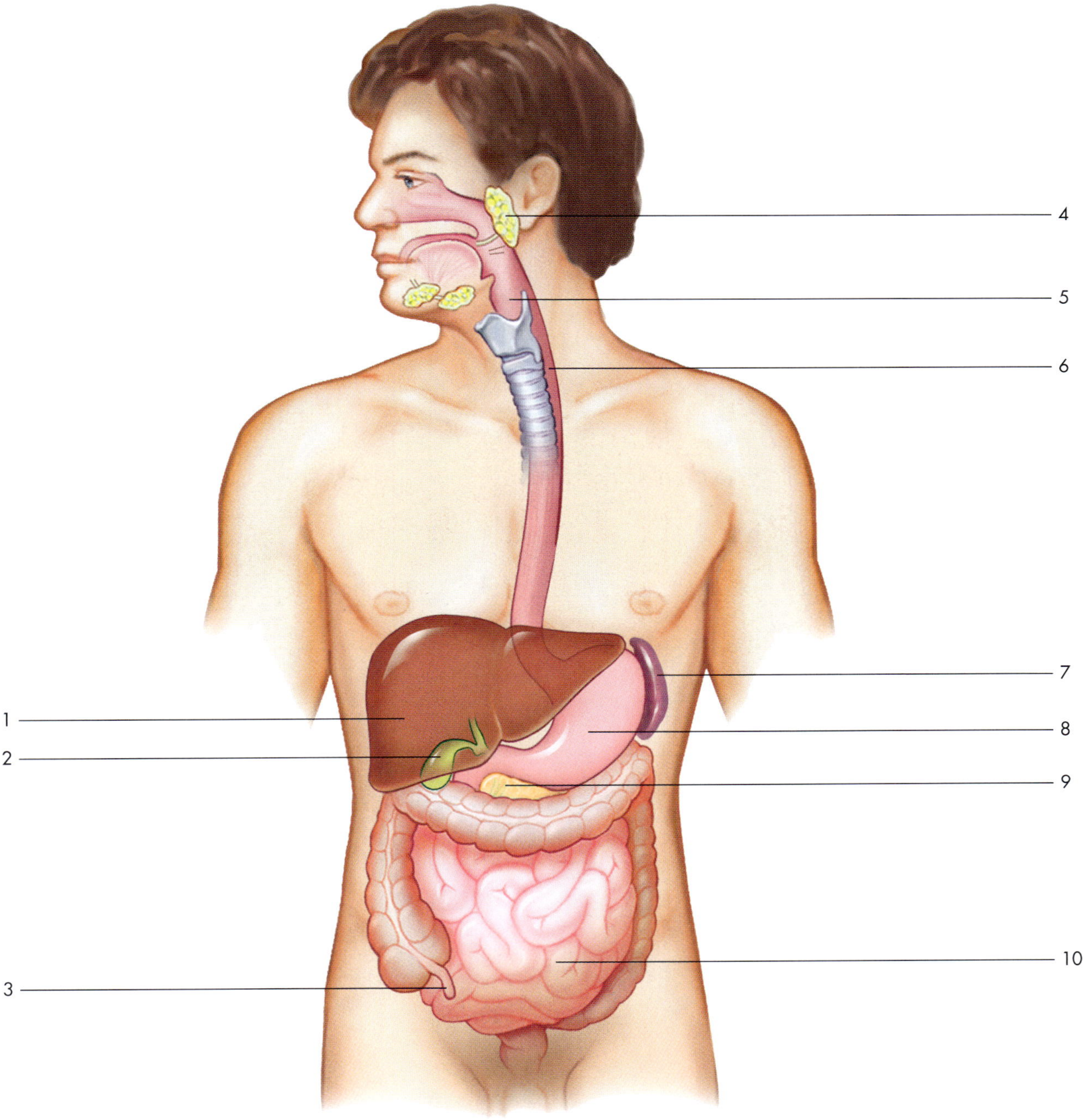

Study and Review II

Word Parts

Prefixes

Give the definitions of the following prefixes.

1. an- ____________________
2. dys- ____________________
3. epi- ____________________
4. hyper- ____________________
5. hypo- ____________________
6. mal- ____________________
7. peri- ____________________
8. post- ____________________
9. dia- ____________________
10. sub- ____________________

Combining Forms

Give the definitions of the following combining forms.

1. amyl/o ____________________
2. append/o ____________________
3. bil/i ____________________
4. bucc/o ____________________
5. celi/o ____________________
6. chol/e ____________________
7. cirrh/o ____________________
8. colon/o ____________________
9. dent/o ____________________
10. enter/o ____________________
11. esophage/o ____________________
12. gastr/o ____________________
13. gingiv/o ____________________
14. gloss/o ____________________
15. hepat/o ____________________
16. ile/o ____________________
17. labi/o ____________________
18. lapar/o ____________________
19. lingu/o ____________________
20. odont/o ____________________
21. prand/i ____________________
22. proct/o ____________________
23. rect/o ____________________
24. stomat/o ____________________

Suffixes

Give the definitions of the following suffixes.

1. -ac ______	**2.** -al ______
3. -algia ______	**4.** -ary ______
5. -ase ______	**6.** -cele ______
7. -oid ______	**8.** -sis ______
9. -ectomy ______	**10.** -emesis ______
11. -form ______	**12.** -genesis ______
13. -ic ______	**14.** -in ______
15. -ion ______	**16.** -ism ______
17. -ist ______	**18.** -itis ______
19. -ive ______	**20.** -logy ______
21. -lysis ______	**22.** -megaly ______
23. -oma ______	**24.** -orexia ______
25. -osis ______	**26.** -rrhea ______
27. -pepsia ______	**28.** -us ______
29. -phagia ______	**30.** -scope ______
31. -scopy ______	**32.** -stalsis ______
33. -stomy ______	**34.** -tomy ______
35. -y ______	**36.** -rrhaphy ______

Identifying Medical Terms

In the spaces provided, write the medical terms for the following meanings.

1. ______ Enzyme that breaks down starch

2. ______ Building up of the body substance in the constructive phase of metabolism

3. ______ Lack of appetite

4. ______ Surgical excision of the appendix

5. ______ Inflammation of the appendix

6. ______________________ Pertaining to bile

7. ______________________ Pertaining to the abdomen

8. ______________________ Difficulty in swallowing

9. ______________________ Inflammation of the liver

10. ______________________ Surgical repair of a hernia

11. ______________________ Pertaining to after meals

12. ______________________ Enlargement of the spleen

13. ______________________ An instrument used in a medical procedure to view the interior of the sigmoid colon

Matching

Select the appropriate lettered meaning for each of the following words.

________	**1.** cirrhosis	**a.** To wash out a cavity
________	**2.** constipation	**b.** To feed liquid or semiliquid food via a tube
________	**3.** diarrhea	**c.** Twisting of the bowel on itself that causes an obstruction
________	**4.** gavage	**d.** Frequent passage of unformed watery stool
________	**5.** hemorrhoid	**e.** Chronic degenerative liver disease
________	**6.** hernia	**f.** Infrequent passage of unduly hard and dry feces
________	**7.** hyperemesis	**g.** Closed sac in the crease of the sacrococcygeal region
________	**8.** lavage	**h.** Abnormal protrusion of an organ or a part of an organ through the wall of the body cavity that normally contains it
________	**9.** pilonidal cyst	**i.** Mass of dilated, tortuous veins in the anorectum
________	**10.** volvulus	**j.** Excessive vomiting
		k. Evacuation of the bowel

Medical Case Snapshots

This learning activity provides an opportunity to relate the medical terminology you are learning to a precise patient case presentation. In the spaces provided, write in your answers.

Case 1

A 54-year-old male was scheduled for a routine visual examination of the colon also known as a ____________. The exam revealed a malignancy of the colon. He was scheduled for a ______________ (a procedure to create a new opening into the colon).

Case 2

A 72-year-old male presents with symptoms of infrequent passage of hard, dry feces. A rectal exam reveals a mass of dilated, tortuous veins in the anorectum. The patient is advised that he has ______________ and ______________. He is to take a laxative to loosen the bowel and is advised to increase his intake of fluids and fiber.

Case 3

A 37-year-old male complains of dull, aching pain in the stomach and back. He has "heartburn and belching." His symptoms suggest peptic ulcer disease, which is often caused by ______________ ______________ (a bacterium). This condition can often be cured with the use of a combination of medications, including ______________ (drugs that kill bacteria).

Study and Review III

Building Medical Terms

Using the following word parts, fill in the blanks to build the correct medical terms.

dys-	-al	-itis
bucc	-ectomy	-cele
gingiv	-osis	
lapar/o	-stomy	

Definition	Medical Term
1. Surgical excision of the appendix	append______
2. Literally means pertaining to the cheek	____________al
3. Chronic degenerative liver disease	cirrh ________
4. The creation of a new opening into the colon	colo_________
5. Inflammation of the diverticula in the colon	diverticul_____
6. Difficulty in digestion; indigestion	_______ pepsia
7. Inflammation of the gums	__________itis
8. Surgical incision into the abdomen	________ tomy
9. Pertaining to the tongue	lingu_________
10. Hernia of part of the rectum into the vagina	recto________

Combining Form Challenge

Using the combining forms provided, write the medical term correctly.

absorpt/o	bil/i	gloss/o
append/o	esophage/o	hepat/o

1. Process by which nutrient material is transferred from the gastrointestinal tract into the bloodstream or lymph: ____________ion

2. Surgical excision of the appendix: ____________ectomy

3. Pertaining to bile: ____________ary

4. Pertaining to the esophagus: _____________ al

5. Partial or total surgical excision of the tongue: ______________ectomy

6. Inflammation of the liver: ____________ itis

Select the Right Term

Select the correct answer, and write it on the line provided.

1. Inflammation of the gallbladder is _______________.

   choledochotomy **cholecystitis** **cheilosis** **appendicitis**

2. Significant accumulation of fluid in the peritoneal cavity is ____________.

   ascites **anabolism** **cirrhosis** **celiac**

3. A surgical procedure that brings one end of the large intestine out through an opening (stoma) made in the abdominal wall is called a _____________.

   colonoscopy **colostomy** **colectomy** **cholecystectomy**

4. The term that means pertaining to the stomach and esophagus is _____________.

   gastroenterology **gastroesophageal** **gastoesophaeal** **gastroenteritis**

5. To feed liquid or semiliquid food via a tube is ________________.

   gastric **enteric** **gavage** **deglutition**

6. Chewing; the physical breaking up of food and mixing with saliva is _______.

   malabsorption **mastication** **lavage** **gavage**

Diagnostic and Laboratory Tests

Select the best answer to each multiple-choice question. Circle the letter of your choice.

1. X-ray examination of the common bile duct, cystic duct, and hepatic ducts.

   a. cholangiography **b.** cholecystography
   c. cholangiopancreatography **d.** ultrasonography

2. Direct visual examination of the colon via a flexible colonoscope.

   a. cholangiography **b.** ultrasonography
   c. fiberoptic colonoscopy **d.** cholecystography

3. Fluoroscopic examination of the esophagus, stomach, and small intestine.

   a. colonoscopy **b.** ultrasonography
   c. cholangiography **d.** gastrointestinal series

4. Endoscopic examination of the esophagus, stomach, and small intestine.

   a. cholangiography **b.** gastroduodenoesophagoscopy
   c. esophagogastroduodenoscopy **d.** gastric analysis

5. Test performed to determine the presence of the hepatitis B virus.

   a. occult blood test **b.** stool culture
   c. hepatitis B surface antigen **d.** ova and parasites test

Abbreviations

Place the correct word, phrase, or abbreviation in the space provided.

1. barium ______________________
2. CHO ______________________
3. HCV ______________________
4. hydrochloric acid ______________________
5. gallbladder ______________________
6. hepatitis A virus ______________________
7. NG ______________________
8. irritable bowel syndrome ______________________
9. postprandial (after meals) ______________________
10. proton-pump inhibitors ______________________

Practical Application

Medical Record Analysis

The Patient Referral Form is an important part of a patient's chart. As part of your learning process and in preparation for a career in a medical environment, you are to assume the role of a medical employee and use the following information—together with your own input—to complete the Patient Referral Form.

PATIENT REFERRAL FORM

Task   Edit   View   Time Scale   Options   Help   Date: 28 September 2017

Patient referred to Seymour Butts, MD, Endoscopy Center, 14 Maddox Drive, Rome, GA 30165, phone number (706) 235-3957, fax (706) 235-8877, for a screening colonoscopy on October 17, 2017, at 8:45 a.m. Advise patient to bring a driver, all current medications, driver's license, and proof of insurance

Referring physician, Angel De'Crohn, MD, Family Practice, 1165 Berry Blvd, Rome, GA 30165, (706) 235-7765, fax (706) 235-6676.

Patient Referral Form

Our practice is affiliated with Mercy Medical Center

Please refer this patient to Mercy Medical Center for any needed surgery or diagnostic procedures so that we can better coordinate this patient's care.

Date: 09/28/17

Patient Name: Ralph J. Starr DOB: 2/24/53 Phone Number 123-456-7890

Appointment Date: ____________________ Time: ____________________

Referred to: ____

____

For:

____________________ Diagnostic Procedure ____________________

____________________ Consultation

____________________ Evaluate and treat, initiating appropriate diagnostic and/or therapeutic services

____________________ Report test results to: ____________________

Reason for referral: ____

Patient Instructions: ____

____

____

Referring Physician's Name: ____________________ Date: ____________________

Phone #: ____________________ Fax #: ____________________

Remit the Record of this Patient's Visit to the Physician Noted Above.

For Office Use Only (appointment made at a time when the patient was not present)

Patient notified of appointment: Date: ____________ Initials: ____________

Unable to contact patient

Attempts to notify: Date/Time/Initials

1. ____
2. ____
3. ____

Comments: ____

Certified Letter Sent: Date: ________________ Initials: ________________

Referral Form Questions

Place the correct answer in the space provided.

1. Write in the Appointment Date: ____________________ Time: ____________________

2. The patient was referred to (write in name of physician, center name, and address):

____

____

____

____

3. The patient was referred for:

_________________________ Diagnostic Procedure

_________________________ Screening Colonoscopy

_________________________ Consultation

_________________________ Evaluate and treat, initiating appropriate diagnostic and/or therapeutic services

_________________________ Report test results to: Angel De'Crohn, MD

4. The Patient Instructions were: _____________________________

5. Write in the name of:

Referring Physician: _____________________________

Date: _________________________________

Phone #: _____________________________

Fax #: ______________________________

Study and Review I

Anatomy and Physiology

Write your answers to the following questions.

1. The cardiovascular system includes:

   a. ______________________ b. ______________________

   c. ______________________ d. ______________________

2. Name the three layers of the heart.

   a. ______________________ b. ______________________

   c. ______________________

3. The heart weighs approximately ______________________ grams.

4. The ______________________ or upper chambers of the heart are separated by the ______________________ septum.

5. The ______________________ or lower chambers of the heart are separated by the ______________________ septum.

6. A/An ______________________ records the heart's electrical activity.

7. The ______________________ ______________________ ______________________ controls the heartbeat.

8. The ______________________ ______________________ is called the *pacemaker of the heart*.

9. Together, the bundle branches and ______________________ comprise the ventricular conduction system.

10. Name the three primary pulse points and state their locations on the body.

    a. ______________________ located ______________________

    b. ______________________ located ______________________

    c. ______________________ located ______________________

11. Define the following terms:

    a. Blood pressure ____

    b. Pulse pressure ____

12. The average adult heart is about the size of a ____________________ and normally beats at a pulse rate of ____________________ to ____________________ beats per minute.

13. A systolic pressure of ____________________ to ____________________ mmHg or a diastolic pressure of ____________________ to ____________________ mmHg is considered "prehypertension" and needs to be monitored on a regular basis.

14. State the primary function of arteries. ____

____

____

15. State the primary function of veins. ____

____

____

ANATOMY LABELING

Identify the structures shown below by filling in the blanks.

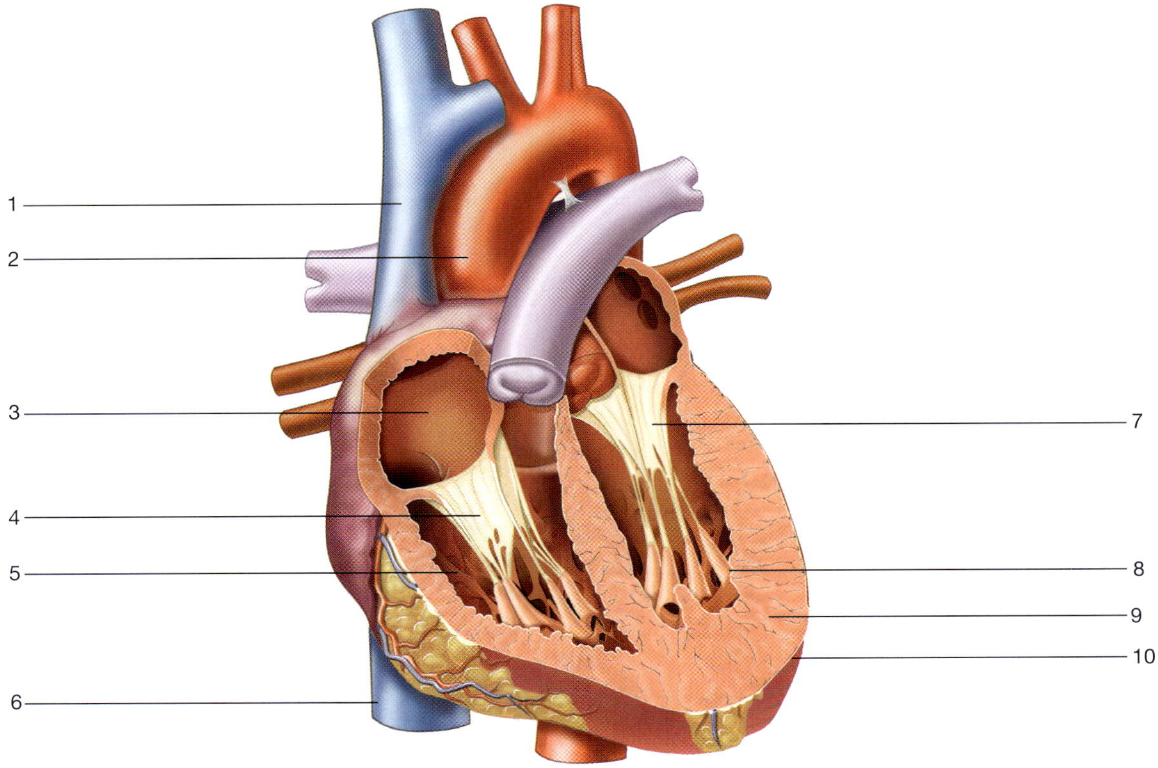

Study and Review II

Word Parts

Prefixes

Give the definitions of the following prefixes.

1. a- ______________________
2. bi- ______________________
3. brady- ______________________
4. con- ______________________
5. end- ______________________
6. endo- ______________________
7. extra- ______________________
8. hyper- ______________________
9. hypo- ______________________
10. peri- ______________________
11. dys- ______________________
12. semi- ______________________
13. tachy- ______________________
14. tri- ______________________

Combining Forms

Give the definitions of the following combining forms.

1. angi/o ______________________
2. arteri/o ______________________
3. ather/o ______________________
4. cardi/o ______________________
5. cyan/o ______________________
6. dilat/o ______________________
7. ech/o ______________________
8. embol/o ______________________
9. hem/o ______________________
10. isch/o ______________________
11. lipid/o ______________________
12. lun/o ______________________
13. man/o ______________________
14. mitr/o ______________________
15. occlus/o ______________________
16. oxy ______________________
17. palpit/o ______________________
18. phleb/o ______________________
19. scler/o ______________________
20. sin/o ______________________
21. steth/o ______________________
22. thromb/o ______________________
23. vas/o ______________________
24. ven/o ______________________

Suffixes

Give the definitions of the following suffixes.

1. -ac ______________________
2. -al ______________________
3. -ar, -ary ______________________
4. -centesis ______________________
5. -metry ______________________
6. -ectasis ______________________
7. -ectomy ______________________
8. -emia ______________________
9. -er ______________________
10. -gen ______________________
11. -graphy ______________________
12. -ia ______________________
13. -ic ______________________
14. -ide ______________________
15. -ion ______________________
16. -ism ______________________
17. -ist ______________________
18. -itis ______________________
19. -ive ______________________
20. -logy ______________________
21. -malacia ______________________
22. -megaly ______________________
23. -meter ______________________
24. -oma ______________________
25. -or ______________________
26. -osis ______________________
27. -pathy ______________________
28. -plasty ______________________
29. -scope ______________________
30. -spasm ______________________
31. -tomy ______________________
32. -um ______________________

Identifying Medical Terms

In the spaces provided, write the medical terms for the following meanings.

1. ______________________ Tumor of a blood vessel
2. ______________________ Surgical repair of a blood vessel(s)
3. ______________________ Pathological condition of narrowing of a blood vessel
4. ______________________ Irregularity or loss (lack of) rhythm of the heartbeat
5. ______________________ Inflammation of an artery
6. ______________________ Valve with two cusps; pertaining to the mitral valve
7. ______________________ Physician who specializes in the study of the heart

8. ______________________________ Enlargement of the heart

9. ______________________________ Pertaining to the heart and lungs

10. ______________________________ Process of drawing together as in the narrowing of a vessel

11. ______________________________ Condition in which a blood clot obstructs a blood vessel

12. ______________________________ Literally means *inflammation of a vein*

13. ______________________________ Rapid heartbeat

14. ______________________________ Medicine that acts directly on smooth muscle cells within blood vessels to make them widen (dilate)

Matching

Select the appropriate lettered meaning for each of the following words.

_____________ **1.** cholesterol

_____________ **2.** claudication

_____________ **3.** dysrhythmia

_____________ **4.** diastole

_____________ **5.** fibrillation

_____________ **6.** lipoprotein

_____________ **7.** cardioversion

_____________ **8.** palpitation

_____________ **9.** percutaneous transluminal coronary angioplasty

_____________ **10.** systole

a. Medical procedure used to treat cardiac arrhythmias

b. Quivering of muscle fiber

c. Fat and protein molecules that are bound together

d. A normal, soft, waxy substance found among the lipids (fats) in the bloodstream and all body cells

e. Literally means *process of lameness, limping*

f. An abnormality of the rhythm or rate of the heartbeat

g. Relaxation phase of the heart cycle

h. Contraction phase of the heart cycle

i. An abnormal rapid throbbing or fluttering of the heart

j. Use of a balloon-tipped catheter to compress fatty plaques against an artery wall

k. Process of being closed

Medical Case Snapshots

This learning activity provides an opportunity to relate the medical terminology you are learning to a precise patient case presentation. In the spaces provided, write in your answers.

Case 1

A 45-year-old male describes experiencing a "squeezing" sensation in his chest during a workout session. This condition, described as __________ ________, occurs when diseased blood vessels restrict blood flow to the heart, causing chest pain that can radiate to the ________ and ________, or to the left arm.

Case 2

A 72-year-old male is diagnosed with arteriosclerotic heart disease (ASHD). Upon ________________ (assessment using a stethoscope to listen to sounds), Dr. Chung hears a bruit or sound of arterial origin. Two conditions often associated with ASHD are ______________ (hardening of the arteries) and ________________ (buildup of fatty substances with subsequent hardening of the arterial walls).

Case 3

The patient is a 62-year-old male experiencing __________ __________ (chest pain). He states that the pain radiates to his neck, jaw, and left arm. An ultrafast CT scan was ordered. After the results of this test were studied, a _____________ ______________ bypass graft (CABG) was discussed with the patient and his wife.

Study and Review III

Building Medical Terms

Using the following word parts, fill in the blanks to build the correct medical terms.

bi-	steth/o	-gen
occlus	veni	-cuspid
sept	-ion	-plasty

Definition	Medical Term
1. Valve with two cusps; pertaining to the mitral valve	_______ cuspid
2. Literally means *process of lameness or limping*	claudicat _____
3. A blockage in a vessel, canal, or passage of the body	__________ ion
4. Colorless, odorless, tasteless gas essential to respiration	oxy _________
5. An abnormal rapid throbbing or fluttering of the heart	palpitat ______
6. Wall or partition that divides a body space or cavity	__________ um
7. Medical instrument used to listen to sounds of the heart	________ scope
8. Valve with three cusps	tri __________
9. Surgical repair of a cardiac valve	valvulo _______
10. Puncture of a vein for the removal of blood for analysis	_____ puncture

Combining Form Challenge

Using the combining forms provided, write the medical term correctly.

angi/o	ather/o	cyan/o
arteri/o	cardi/o	phleb/o

1. Surgical repair of a blood vessel: ________plasty

2. Pertaining to an artery: _______al

3. Tumor of an artery containing a fatty substance: _________oma

4. Enlargement of the heart: ___________megaly

5. The skin, fingernails, and mucous membranes can appear slightly blue: ___________osis

6. Literally means *inflammation of a vein*: ________itis

Select the Right Term

Select the correct answer, and write it on the line provided.

1. Abnormally slow heartbeat defined as less than 60 beats per minute is ______________.

   bruit **cardioversion** **bradycardia** **tachycardia**

2. Abnormal high levels of lipids in the blood is ______________.

   hyperlipidemia **hyperlipdemia** **hypolipidemia** **hypolipdemia**

3. Pertaining to the sac surrounding the heart is ______________.

   pericardial **pericardiocentesis** **pericarditis** **phlebitis**

4. Valves of the aorta and pulmonary artery; shaped like a crescent is ______________.

   sinoatrial **tricuspid** **bicuspid** **semilunar**

5. Pertains to an organic compound consisting of three molecules of fatty acids is ______________.

   tricuspid **triglyceride** **systole** **triglyeride**

6. Condition in which there is a lack of oxygen due to decreased blood supply to a part of the body caused by constriction or obstruction of a blood vessel is ______________.

   infarction **murmur** **ischemia** **occlusion**

Diagnostic and Laboratory Tests

Select the best answer to each multiple-choice question. Circle the letter of your choice.

1. ______________________________ is an intracardiac procedure that maps the electrical conduction of cardiac arrhythmias.
   a. Electrocardiogram
   b. Electrocardiomyogram
   c. Electrophysiology
   d. Cardiac catheterization

2. Blood tests performed to determine cardiac damage in an acute myocardial infarction.
   a. cardiac enzymes
   b. high-density lipoproteins
   c. triglycerides
   d. low-density lipoproteins

3. Method of recording a patient's ECG for 24 hours.
   a. stress test
   b. Holter monitor
   c. ultrasonography
   d. angiography

4. Test used to visualize an organ or tissue by using high-frequency sound waves.
   - **a.** electrophysiology
   - **b.** stress test
   - **c.** ultrasonography
   - **d.** cholesterol

5. X-ray recording of a blood vessel after the injection of a radiopaque contrast medium.
   - **a.** ultrasonography
   - **b.** angiography
   - **c.** stress test
   - **d.** cardiac catheterization

Abbreviations

Place the correct word, phrase, or abbreviation in the space provided.

1. acute myocardial infarction ______
2. atrioventricular ______
3. BP ______
4. CAD ______
5. cardiac catheterization ______
6. ECG, EKG ______
7. HDL ______
8. heart and lungs ______
9. MI ______
10. tPA, TPA ______

Practical Application

Soap: Chart Note Analysis

This exercise will make you aware of the information, abbreviations, and medical terminology typically found in a cardiology patient's chart. Refer to Appendix III, *Abbreviations and Symbols*.

Read the chart note and answer the questions that follow.

GREENLEAF MEDICAL CENTER

Task Edit View Time Scale Options Help Date: 17 May 2017

420 East First Avenue •Rome, GA 30165 •(123) 456-1234

Cardiology Services

Patient: Moore, William T. **Date:** 05/06/2017 **Patient ID:** 32367

DOB: 3/26/1965 **Age:** 52 **Gender:** Male **Allergies:** NKDA

Provider: David R. Briones, MD

S

Subjective:

Chief Complaint: "Lately I have noticed tightness in my chest during exercise and I feel out of breath. I am real anxious and worried about myself."

52 y/o Caucasian male describes experiencing "tightness" in his chest during a work-out session. Noted patient clenching his fist while describing dyspnea (shortness of breath) and how anxious he felt. He denies nausea, vomiting, or radiating pain to his left arm or jaw. The uncomfortable sensation "just went away" after he stopped exercising. He states that he has no prior history of cardiac disease.

O

Objective:

Vital Signs: T: 98.4 F; **P:** 84; **R:** 20; **BP:** 138/90

Ht: 5′ 11″

Wt: 196 lb

General Appearance: Well-developed and muscular. No obvious signs of physical distress noted such as edema, pallor, or diaphoresis. Overall health appears WNL.

Heart: Rate at 84 beats per minute, rhythm regular, no extra sounds, no murmurs.

Lungs: CTA

Abd: Bowel sounds all four quadrants, no masses or tenderness.

MS: Joints and muscles symmetric; no swelling, masses, or deformity; normal spinal curvature. No tenderness to palpation of joints. Full ROM, movement smooth, no crepitant (crackling) sound heard, no tenderness. Muscle strength: able to maintain flexion against resistance and without tenderness.

A

Assessment:

Chest pain (angina pectoris).

P

Plan:

1. Schedule patient for an EKG and blood enzyme studies ASAP.
2. Start patient on nitroglycerin (coronary vasodilator) sublingual tablets 0.4 mg prn for chest pain. Instruct patient to seek medical attention immediately if pain is not relieved by nitroglycerin tablets, taken one every 5 minutes over a 15-minute period.
3. To return in 2 weeks for follow-up.
4. Discuss family cardiac history as related to HTN, obesity, diabetes, coronary artery disease, and sudden death of any family member occurring at a young age.
5. Educate patient that angina pectoris occurs due to myocardial ischemia that results when cardiac workload and myocardial oxygen demand exceed the ability of the coronary arteries to supply oxygenated blood. This commonly occurs during exercise or other activity.

Chart Note Questions

Place the correct answer in the space provided.

1. Signs and symptoms of angina pectoris include tightness in the chest, apprehension, and shortness of breath, which is also called ______________________.

2. A complete physical, an EKG, and ______________________ studies are important in determining the diagnosis of angina pectoris.

3. Myocardial ischemia is a result of the body's inability to supply ______________________ blood.

4. EKG is an abbreviation for ______________________.

5. Nitroglycerin is a ______________________ ______________________ used to treat angina pectoris.

Study and Review I

Anatomy and Physiology

Write your answers to the following questions.

1. Name the three formed elements of blood.

   a. ______________________ **b.** ______________________

   c. ______________________

2. State the function of erythrocytes. ______________________

   ____

   ____

3. There are approximately ______________ million erythrocytes per cubic millimeter of blood.

4. The lifespan of an erythrocyte is ______________.

5. State the function of leukocytes. ______________

6. There are approximately ______________ thousand leukocytes per cubic millimeter of blood.

7. Name the five types of leukocytes.

   a. ______________ b. ______________

   c. ______________ d. ______________

   e. ______________

8. State the function of thrombocytes. ______________

9. There are approximately ______________ thrombocytes per cubic millimeter of blood.

10. Name the four blood types.

   a. ______________ b. ______________

   c. ______________ d. ______________

11. State the three main functions of the lymphatic system.

   a. ______________

   b. ______________

   c. ______________

12. Name the three accessory organs of the lymphatic system.

   a. ______________

   b. ______________

   c. ______________

ANATOMY LABELING

Identify the structures shown below by filling in the blanks.

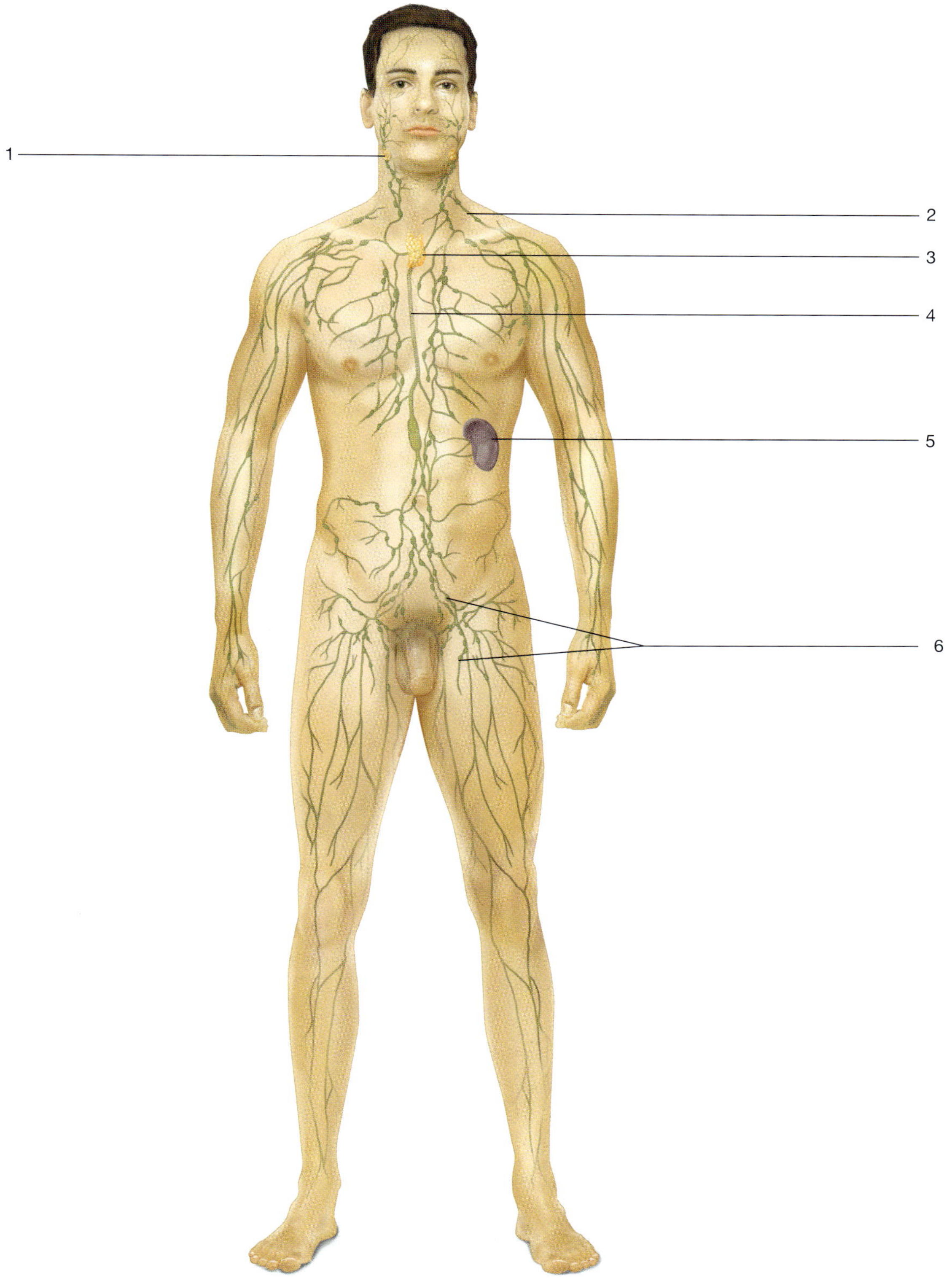

Study and Review II

Word Parts

Prefixes

Give the definitions of the following prefixes.

1. an- ________________
2. anti- ________________
3. auto- ________________
4. ana- ________________
5. extra- ________________
6. hyper- ________________
7. hypo- ________________
8. mono- ________________
9. pan- ________________
10. poly- ________________
11. pro- ________________
12. trans- ________________
13. hyp- ________________

Combining Forms

Give the definitions of the following combining forms.

1. agglutin/o ________________
2. angi/o ________________
3. anis/o ________________
4. bas/o ________________
5. chromat/o ________________
6. coagul/o ________________
7. cyt/o ________________
8. eosin/o ________________
9. erythr/o ________________
10. glyc/o ________________
11. hemat/o ________________
12. hem/o ________________
13. immun/o ________________
14. leuk/o ________________
15. lymph/o ________________
16. macr/o ________________
17. neutr/o ________________
18. plasm/o ________________
19. septic/o ________________
20. ser/o ________________
21. sider/o ________________
22. splen/o ________________
23. thym/o ________________
24. vascul/o ________________

Suffixes

Give the definitions of the following suffixes.

1. -able ______________________
2. -ant ______________________
3. -apheresis ______________________
4. -blast ______________________
5. -body ______________________
6. -edema ______________________
7. -culture ______________________
8. -cyte ______________________
9. -ectomy ______________________
10. -emia ______________________
11. -ergy ______________________
12. -gen ______________________
13. -phylaxis ______________________
14. -globin ______________________
15. -ic ______________________
16. -in ______________________
17. -ion ______________________
18. -ist ______________________
19. -itis ______________________
20. -logy ______________________
21. -lysis ______________________
22. -megaly ______________________
23. -oma ______________________
24. -osis ______________________
25. -penia ______________________
26. -phil ______________________
27. -poiesis ______________________
28. -rrhage ______________________
29. -stasis ______________________
30. -tomy ______________________
31. -ia ______________________
32. -oxia ______________________

Identifying Medical Terms

In the spaces provided, write the medical terms for the following meanings.

1. ______________________ Process of clumping together, as of blood cells that are incompatible
2. ______________________ An individual hypersensitivity to a substance that is usually harmless
3. ______________________ Protein substance produced in the body in response to an invading foreign substance
4. ______________________ Substance that works against the formation of blood clots
5. ______________________ Invading foreign substance that induces the formation of antibodies
6. ______________________ Process of infusing a patient's own blood
7. ______________________ Capable of forming a clot

8. ______________________ Excess of creatine in the blood

9. ______________________ Blood clot carried in the bloodstream

10. ______________________ Granular leukocyte

11. ______________________ Literally means *one who specializes in the study of the blood*

12. ______________________ Blood protein; the iron-containing pigment of red blood cells

13. ______________________ Pathological condition of excessive amounts of sugar in the blood

14. ______________________ Pathological condition of excessive amounts of lipids (fat) in the blood

15. ______________________ White blood cell

16. ______________________ Control or stopping of the flow of lymph

17. ______________________ Condition of excessive amounts of mononuclear leukocytes in the blood

18. ______________________ Chemical substance that interacts with calcium salts to produce thrombin

19. ______________________ Abnormal enlargement of the spleen

20. ______________________ Clotting cell; blood platelet

Matching

Select the appropriate lettered meaning for each of the following words.

_________ **1.** autotransfusion

_________ **2.** erythrocyte

_________ **3.** erythropoietin

_________ **4.** extravasation

_________ **5.** hemorrhage

_________ **6.** immunoglobulin

_________ **7.** hemochromatosis

_________ **8.** radioimmunoassay

_________ **9.** reticulocyte

_________ **10.** thrombectomy

a. Method of determining the concentration of protein-bound hormones in the blood plasma

b. Genetic disease condition in which iron is not metabolized properly and accumulates in body tissues

c. Blood protein capable of acting as an antibody

d. Mature red blood cell that does not contain a nucleus

e. Hormone that stimulates the production of red blood cells

f. Literally means bursting forth of blood; bleeding

g. Process by which fluids and/or medications escape from the blood vessel into surrounding tissue

h. Process of infusing a patient's own blood

i. Surgical excision of a blood clot

j. Red blood cell containing a network of granules

k. White blood cell

Medical Case Snapshots

This learning activity provides an opportunity to relate the medical terminology you are learning to a precise patient case presentation. In the spaces provided, write in your answers.

Case 1

A 52-year-old female states, "It was months after the death of my husband when I began dating a younger man. We became sexually involved. I am so afraid. Bill has just told me that he is HIV positive and could have AIDS." AIDS is a disease caused by the ______ _____________ virus which invades the ______ lymphocytes.

Case 2

A 15-year-old female complains of being tired, experiencing dizziness, headaches, fast heartbeat, and shortness of breath (_____). A possible diagnosis is anemia. The symptoms of anemia are due to a deficient amount of oxygen in the blood known as ____________. Bloodwork is ordered and the patient is to return in 2 weeks.

Case 3

Two weeks after the initial exam, the 15-year-old female was seen by Dr. Mann. The diagnosis of anemia was confirmed. With anemia special attention is given to the amount of _____________ (or iron-containing pigment of red blood cells) and the percentage of solid components compared to the liquid components of blood called __________. The patient was prescribed an antianemic agent that is used to treat iron-deficiency anemia.

Study and Review III

Building Medical Terms

Using the following word parts, fill in the blanks to build the correct medical terms.

mono-	sider/o	-culture
erythr/o	thromb	-megaly
hem/o	-in	
lymph	-cyte	

Definition	Medical Term
1. Formation of red blood cells	_______poiesis
2. Plasma protein found in body fluids and cells	globul_______
3. Destruction of red blood cells	_________lysis
4. Red blood cell containing a network of granules	reticulo_______
5. Lymphoid neoplasm, usually malignant	_________oma
6. Red blood cell	_________cyte
7. Bacterial culture of blood	sero________
8. Lack of iron in the blood	________penia
9. Abnormal enlargement of the spleen	spleno_______
10. Formation of a blood clot within the vascular system	_________osis

Combining Form Challenge

Using the combining forms provided, write the medical term correctly.

hem/o	erythr/o	leuk/o
coagul/o	hemat/o	lymph/o

1. Destruction of red blood cells _______ lysis

2. Capable of forming a clot: ______able

3. Immature red blood cell that is found only in bone marrow: ______blast

4. Literally means *study of the blood*: __________ logy

5. Disease of the blood characterized by overproduction of leukocytes: _____ emia

6. Abnormal accumulation of lymph in the interstitial spaces: _______edema

Select the Right Term

Select the correct answer, and write it on the line provided.

1. An individual hypersensitivity to a substance that is usually harmless is _______.

   anaphylaxis **anemia** **AIDS** **allergy**

2. Protein substance produced in the body in response to an invading foreign substance is ___________.

   antigen **antibody** **albumin** **fibrinogen**

3. Hereditary blood disease characterized by prolonged coagulation and tendency to bleed is _______________.

   hemophilia **hemolysis** **hemorrhage** **hemochromatosis**

4. Hereditary anemia occurring in populations bordering the Mediterranean Sea and in Southeast Asia is _______________.

   hemolytic **pernicious** **thalassemia** **sickle cell**

5. Blood clot carried in the bloodstream is _____________.

   thrombus **coagulable** **extravasation** **embolus**

6. Essential factor in the production of thrombin and blood clotting is __________.

   thrombin **thromboplastin** **thrombocyte** **prothrombin**

Diagnostic and Laboratory Tests

Select the best answer to each multiple-choice question. Circle the letter of your choice.

1. Blood test to identify antigen–antibody reactions.
   a. erythrocyte sedimentation rate
   b. hematocrit
   c. immunoglobulins
   d. antinuclear antibodies

2. Blood test that includes a hematocrit, hemoglobin, red and white blood cell count, and differential.
   a. blood typing
   b. sedimentation rate
   c. CBC
   d. Hb, Hgb

3. Blood test performed on whole blood to determine the percentage of red blood cells in the total blood volume.
   a. RBC
   b. WBC
   c. Hct
   d. PTT

4. Blood test to determine the number of leukocytes present.
   a. RBC
   b. WBC
   c. Hct
   d. PTT

5. Puncture of the earlobe or forearm to determine the time required for blood to stop flowing.
   a. bleeding time
   b. platelet count
   c. prothrombin time
   d. PTT

Abbreviations

Place the correct word, phrase, or abbreviation in the space provided.

1. acquired immunodeficiency syndrome ______
2. acute lymphocytic leukemia ______
3. CML ______
4. hemoglobin ______
5. Hct ______
6. human immunodeficiency virus ______
7. PJP ______
8. PT ______
9. RBC ______
10. radioimmunoassay ______

Practical Application

Medical Record Analysis

This exercise contains information, abbreviations, and medical terminology from an actual medical record or case study that has been adapted for this text. The names and any personal information have been created by the author. Read and study each form or case study and then answer the questions that follow. You may refer to Appendix III, *Abbreviations and Symbols*.

HARBIN CLINIC HEMATOLOGY

Task Edit View Time Scale Options Help Date: 17 May 2017

2324 Shorter Avenue
Rome, GA 30165
(706) 555-1234

Patient: Sanchez, Carlos
100 Main Street
Cedar Bluff, AL 35959

Age/DOB: 49 yrs 19 Feb. 1968
Home: (256) 123-4567

Results

Lab Accession # 0010871292009
Ordering Provider: Mann, Keith
Performing Location: Main Harbin Clinic

Collected: 4/20/17 10:38:00 AM
Resulted: 4/21/17 10:20:00 AM
Verified By: Mann, Keith
Auto Verify: N
Stage: Final

CBC with Auto Differential Count (diff)

Test	Result	Units	Flag	Reference Range
WBC	7.9	$\times 10^3/\mu L$		4.8–10.8
RBC	4.44	$\times 10^3/\mu L$	L	4.6–6.13
HGB	14.4	g/dL		14.1–18.1
HCT	41.9	%	L	43.5–53.7
MCV	94.0	fL		80.0–99.0
MCH	35.4	Pg	H	26.0–34.0
MCHC	34.3	g/dL		33.0–37.0
RDW	12.6	%		11.6–14.8
PLATELETS	248	$\times 10^3/\mu L$		130–400
MPV	8.8	fL		7.4–10.4
NEUT%	56.3	%		37.0–80.0

Test	Result	Units	Flag	Reference Range
LYMPH%	32.4	%		10.0–50.0
MONO%	8.2	%		0.1–10.0
EOS%	1.6	%		0.1–6.0
BASO%	1.5	%		0.0–3.0
NEUT#	4.5	$\times 10^3/\mu L$		2.9–6.2
LYMPH#	2.6	$\times 10^3/\mu L$		0.8–3.9
MONO#	0.7	$\times 10^3/\mu L$		0.0–1.2
EOS#	0.1	$\times 10^3/\mu L$		0.0–0.6
BASO#	0.1	$\times 10^3/\mu L$		0.1–0.3

Medical Record Questions

Place the correct answer in the space provided.

1. What does the abbreviation *CBC* mean? ______________________
2. What does the abbreviation *diff* mean? ______________________
3. Which one of the test results was flagged high? ______________________
4. What is the normal range for white blood cells? ______________________
5. What is the normal range for red blood cells? ______________________

Study and Review I

Anatomy and Physiology

Write your answers to the following questions.

1. List the organs of the respiratory system.

a. ______________________ **b.** ______________________

c. ______________________ **d.** ______________________

e. ______________________ **f.** ______________________

2. State the primary function of the respiratory system.

____

____

3. Define external respiration ______________________

4. Define internal respiration ______________________

5. List the five functions of the nose.

a. ______________________ **b.** ______________________

c. ______________________ **d.** ______________________

e. ______________________

6. List the three functions of the pharynx.

a. ______________________ **b.** ______________________

c. ______________________

7. State the function of the epiglottis ______________________

8. Define glottis ______________________

9. State the function of the larynx ______________________

10. State the function of the trachea ______________________

11. State the function of the bronchi ______________________

12. Give a brief description of the lungs ______________________

13. Define pleura ______________________

14. The thoracic cavity is separated from the abdominal cavity by a musculomembranous wall commonly known as the ______________________

15. The central portion of the thoracic cavity between the lungs is a space called the ______________________

16. The right lung has _________________________ lobes and the left lung has _________________________ lobes.

17. The air cells of the lungs are the ____

18. State the main function of the lungs ____

19. The vital signs, which are essential elements for determining an individual's state of health, are _________________________, _________________________, ________________________________, and

____

20. Define the following terms:

a. Tidal volume ____

b. Residual volume ____

c. Vital capacity ____

21. The ____________________ ____________________ and the ____________________ of the central nervous system regulate and control respiration.

22. The normal resting respiratory rate for a newborn is __________________ to __________________breaths per minute.

23. The normal resting respiratory rate for an adult is ______________________________ to

______________________________ breaths per minute.

ANATOMY LABELING

Identify the structures shown below by filling in the blanks.

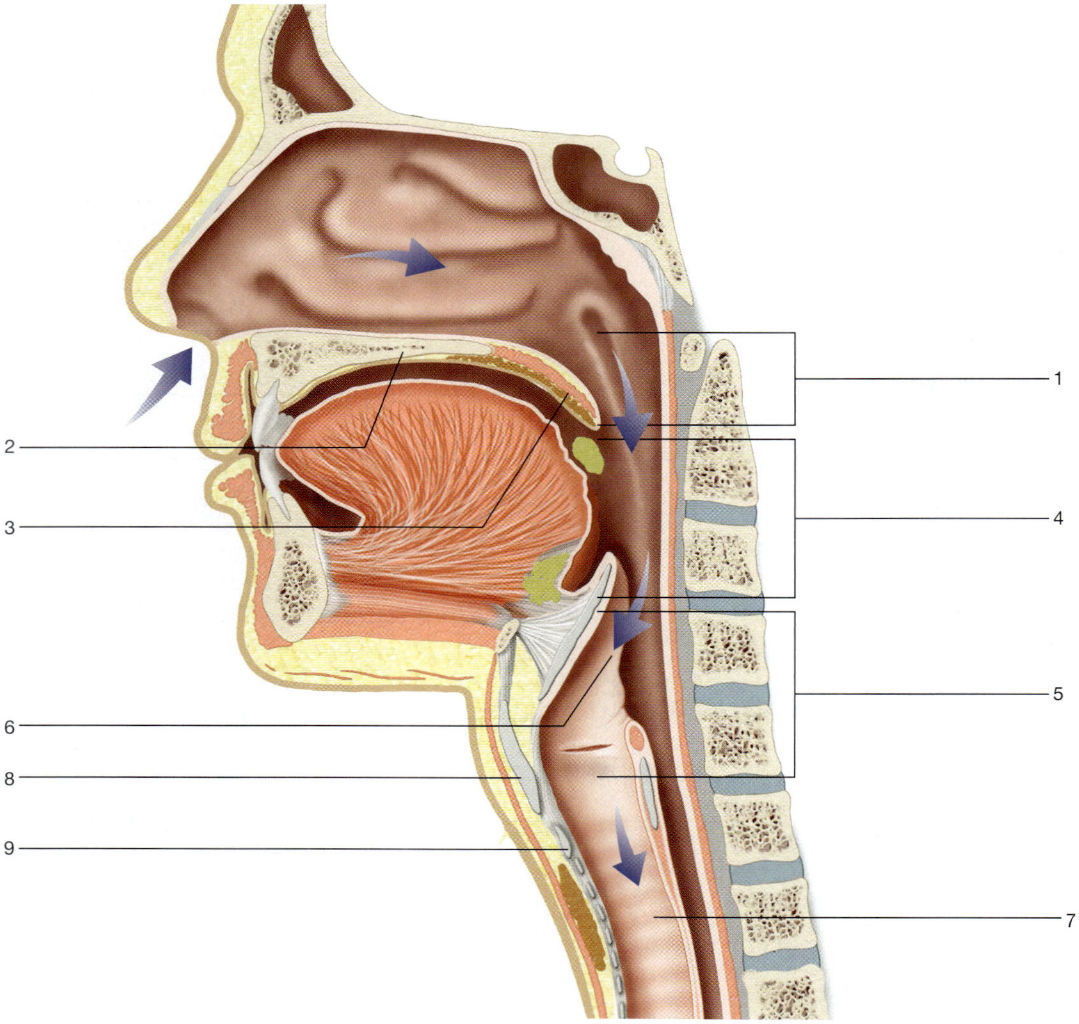

Study and Review II

Word Parts

Prefixes

Give the definitions of the following prefixes.

1. a- ______________________
2. epi- ______________________
3. dys- ______________________
4. endo- ______________________
5. eu- ______________________
6. ex- ______________________
7. hyp- ______________________
8. hyper- ______________________
9. in- ______________________
10. tachy- ______________________

Combining Forms

Give the definitions of the following combining forms.

1. alveol/o ______________________
2. anthrac/o ______________________
3. atel/o ______________________
4. bronch/o ______________________
5. coni/o ______________________
6. halat/o ______________________
7. laryng/o ______________________
8. nas/o ______________________
9. olfact/o ______________________
10. or/o ______________________
11. orth/o ______________________
12. pector/o ______________________
13. pharyng/o ______________________
14. pleur/o ______________________
15. pneum/o ______________________
16. py/o ______________________
17. rhin/o ______________________
18. rhonch/o ______________________
19. spir/o ______________________
20. thorac/o ______________________
21. tonsill/o ______________________
22. trache/o ______________________
23. tubercul/o ______________________

Suffixes

Give the definitions of the following suffixes.

1. -al ______________________
2. -algia ______________________
3. -centesis ______________________
4. -dynia ______________________
5. -ectasis ______________________
6. -ectomy ______________________
7. -ic ______________________
8. -ia ______________________
9. -ion ______________________
10. -itis ______________________
11. -meter ______________________
12. -osis ______________________
13. -oma ______________________
14. -staxis ______________________
15. -plasty ______________________
16. -or ______________________
17. -pnea ______________________
18. -ptysis ______________________
19. -rrhea ______________________
20. -scope ______________________
21. -stomy ______________________
22. -tomy ______________________
23. -us ______________________

Identifying Medical Terms

In the spaces provided, write the medical terms for the following meanings.

1. ______________________ Pertaining to a small air sac in the lungs
2. ______________________ Chronic dilation of a bronchus or bronchi
3. ______________________ Inflammation of the bronchi
4. ______________________ Condition of difficulty in speaking
5. ______________________ Good or normal breathing
6. ______________________ Spitting up blood
7. ______________________ Process of breathing in
8. ______________________ Inflammation of the larynx
9. ______________________ A collection of air between the chest wall and lungs
10. ______________________ Surgical repair of the nose
11. ______________________ Discharge from the nose
12. ______________________ Inflammation of a sinus

Matching

Select the appropriate lettered meaning for each of the following words.

_____________ **1.** cough

_____________ **2.** cystic fibrosis

_____________ **3.** influenza

_____________ **4.** inhalation

_____________ **5.** olfaction

_____________ **6.** pleurodynia

_____________ **7.** rhinovirus

_____________ **8.** sputum

_____________ **9.** tachypnea

_____________ **10.** thoracentesis

a. Substance coughed up from the lungs

b. Pain in the pleura

c. Process of smelling

d. One of a subgroup of viruses that causes the common cold in humans

e. Rapid breathing

f. Process of breathing in

g. Surgical puncture of the chest wall for removal of fluid

h. Sudden, forceful expulsion of air from the lungs

i. Inherited disease that affects the pancreas, respiratory system, and sweat glands

j. Slow breathing

k. Acute, contagious respiratory infection caused by a virus

Medical Case Snapshots

This learning activity provides an opportunity to relate the medical terminology you are learning to a precise patient case presentation. In the spaces provided, write in your answers.

Case 1

A 7-year-old male is seen in the emergency room with wheezing, dyspnea, and a feeling of constriction in the chest. He is experiencing an acute exacerbation of ______________. The ER personnel find that he has an inability to breathe unless he is upright. This condition is called ______________ and he is placed in a sitting position. See Figure 11.7.

Case 2

A 58-year-old male presents with ______________ (difficulty in breathing), _________ ___ _________ (abbreviated SOB), fatigue, and wheezing. A smoker for 40 years, he has had bronchitis several times during the past 5 years. With the use of a ______________ (instrument for measuring lung volume), it was determined that he had emphysema or COPD, an abbreviation for ______________ ______________ ______________ ____________.

Case 3

A 28-year-old male returns to the clinic for a follow-up visit after being diagnosed with _____________ (an infectious disease caused by the tubercle bacillus). The lab performs a ___________ culture (to determine the presence of pathogenic microorganisms).

Study and Review III

Building Medical Terms

Using the following word parts, fill in the blanks to build the correct medical terms.

dys-	thorac/o	-pnea
pharyng	-ectasis	-ectomy
rhin/o	-staxis	-osis

Definition	Medical Term
1. The collapse of an alveolus, a lobule, or a larger lung unit	atel ___________
2. Literally means *difficulty in breathing*	_________ pnea
3. Nosebleed	epi __________
4. Abnormally deep and rapid breathing	hyper ________
5. Inflammation of the pharynx	___________ itis
6. Surgical excision of the left or right lung	pneumon ____

(*continued*)

Definition	Medical Term
7. Surgical repair of the nose	________ plasty
8. Rapid breathing	tachy ________
9. Incision into the chest wall	________ tomy
10. Infectious disease caused by the tubercle bacillus	tubercul _____

Combining Form Challenge

Using the combining forms provided, write the medical term correctly.

anthrac/o	hem/o	olfact/o
bronch/o	laryng/o	orth/o

1. Lung condition caused by inhalation of coal dust and silica: ________osis

2. Medical instrument used to visually examine the bronchi: _______scope

3. Spitting up blood: _______ptysis

4. Medical instrument used to visually examine the larynx: ___________ scope

5. Process of smelling: _________ion

6. Inability to breathe unless in an upright or straight position: ________ pnea

Select the Right Term

Select the correct answer, and write it on the line provided.

1. Disease of the bronchi characterized by wheezing and dyspnea is _______________.

anthracosis **asphyxia** **asthma** **atelectasis**

2. Acute respiratory disease characterized by a barking cough is _________________.

cough **croup** **cystic fibrosis** **dysphonia**

3. Condition of deficient amounts of oxygen in the inspired air is _________________.

eupnea **hyperpnea** **hypoxia** **inhalation**

4. Acute, infectious disease characterized by a cough with a "whooping" sound is __________.

laryngitis **pneumonia** **pharyngitis** **pertussis**

5. Abnormal sound heard on auscultation of the chest; a crackling sound is _____________.

rale **rhonchus** **stridor** **wheeze**

6. One of the subgroup of viruses that causes the common cold is __________________.

syncytial **rhinovirus** **rhinorrhea** **influenza**

Diagnostic and Laboratory Tests

Select the best answer to each multiple-choice question. Circle the letter of your choice.

1. Test performed on sputum to detect the presence of *Mycobacterium tuberculosis*.
   a. antistreptolysin O titer
   b. acid-fast bacilli
   c. pulmonary function test
   d. bronchoscopy

2. Visual examination of the nasal passages.
   a. bronchoscopy
   b. laryngoscopy
   c. rhinoscopy
   d. rhinoplasty

3. ______________________________ is/are important in determining respiratory acidosis and/or alkalosis and metabolic acidosis and/or alkalosis.
   a. Acid-fast bacilli
   b. Antistreptolysin O titer
   c. Arterial blood gases
   d. Pulmonary function test

4. Series of tests to determine the diffusion of oxygen and carbon dioxide across the cell membrane in the lungs.
   a. acid-fast bacilli
   b. antistreptolysin O titer
   c. arterial blood gases
   d. pulmonary function test

5. Visual examination of the larynx, trachea, and bronchi via a flexible scope.
   a. bronchoscopy
   b. laryngoscopy
   c. laryngoscope
   d. rhinoscopy

Abbreviations

Place the correct word, phrase, or abbreviation in the space provided.

1. acid-fast bacilli ______________________________
2. CF ______________________________
3. chest x-ray ______________________________
4. chronic obstructive pulmonary disease ______________________________
5. ET ______________________________
6. hyaline membrane disease ______________________________
7. respiration ______________________________
8. SARS ______________________________
9. shortness of breath ______________________________
10. TB ______________________________

Practical Application

Medical Record Analysis

This exercise contains information, abbreviations, and medical terminology from an actual medical record or case study that has been adapted for this text. The names and any personal information have been created by the author. Read and study each form or case study and then answer the questions that follow. You may refer to Appendix III, *Abbreviations and Symbols*.

GOODWILL HEALTH CLINIC

Task Edit View Time Scale Options Help Date: 17 May 2017

1001 Evergreen Park Drive • Lakeland, FL 33813 • (123) 456-7890

Progress Note

Wilmer Sanchez, Patient # 8234

May 17, 2017

S Subjective:

The patient presents today for reevaluation.

Wilmer Sanchez is a 28-year-old male migrant worker seen in the Lakeland, FL, office. Patient presents with a history of pulmonary tuberculosis and returns for a check of his sputum and a liver function test. He has been taking isoniazid, rifampin, and ethambutol for 4 months. He states that since he has been taking his medicine, he is feeling better.

O Objective:

The patient appears to be in no apparent distress. The patient's mood and affect appeared normal throughout the visit. The patient is afebrile, without fever, P 72, R 18, BP 118/64, Wt 143. No rales noted upon auscultation. Occasional cough, nonproductive.

A Assessment:

Apparent state of health improved over the last 4 months. Patient has gained 3 lbs.

Patient is following medication regimen and does participate in the directly observed therapy (DOT) system, which is documented in his record.

P Plan:

Send to lab for a sputum culture and liver function test.

Schedule a return visit for 2 weeks.

Medical Record Questions

Place the correct answer in the space provided.

1. Define rale. ______________________________
2. What does the abbreviation *DOT* mean? ______________________________
3. Define afebrile. ______________________________
4. Did this patient seem anxious? ______________________________
5. What type of cough did this patient have? ______________________________

Study and Review I

Anatomy and Physiology

Write your answers to the following questions.

1. List the organs of the urinary system.

a. ______________________ **b.** ______________________

c. ______________________ **d.** ______________________

2. State the vital function of the urinary system. ______________________

____

3. Define hilum. ______________________

4. Define renal pelvis. ______________________

5. The medulla is the ______________________ portion of the kidney.

6. Define nephron. ______________________

7. Each nephron consists of a ______________________ and a ______________________.

8. The renal corpuscle consists of ______________________ and ______________________.

9. Urine is formed by the process of ______________________ and ______________________ in the nephron.

10. An average of ______________________ to ______________________ mL of urine is voided daily.

11. Describe the ureters and state their function. ______________________

____

12. Describe the urinary bladder and state its function. ______________________

____

13. The external urinary opening is the ______________________.

14. Define urinalysis. ______________________

____

15. Give the normal constituents for the physical examination of urine.

a. Color ______________________________

b. Appearance ______________________________

c. Reaction ______________________________

d. Specific gravity ______________________________

e. Odor ______________________________

f. Quantity ______________________________

16. A urine that has a fruity, sweet odor can indicate ______________________________

______________________________.

17. Under chemical examination, the presence of protein in urine is an important sign of ______________________________

______________________________.

ANATOMY LABELING

Identify the structures shown below by filling in the blanks.

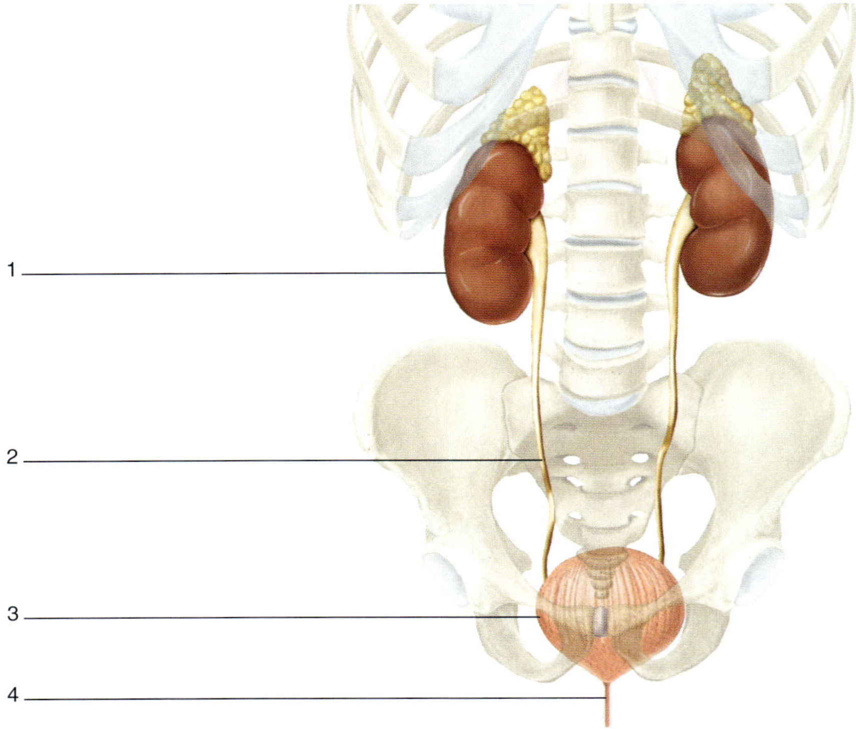

Study and Review II

Word Parts

Prefixes

Give the definitions of the following prefixes.

1. an- ______________________
2. anti- ______________________
3. dia- ______________________
4. dys- ______________________
5. en- ______________________
6. hydro- ______________________
7. extra- ______________________
8. in- ______________________
9. olig- ______________________
10. per- ______________________
11. ultra- ______________________
12. poly- ______________________

Combining Forms

Give the definitions of the following combining forms.

1. albumin/o ______________________
2. bacter/i ______________________
3. calc/i ______________________
4. corpore/o ______________________
5. cyst/o ______________________
6. excret/o ______________________
7. glomerul/o ______________________
8. glycos/o ______________________
9. hemat/o ______________________
10. keton/o ______________________
11. lith/o ______________________
12. meat/o ______________________
13. micturit/o ______________________
14. nephr/o ______________________
15. noct/o ______________________
16. perine/o ______________________
17. peritone/o ______________________
18. pyel/o ______________________
19. ren/o ______________________
20. son/o ______________________
21. ur/o ______________________
22. ureter/o ______________________
23. urethr/o ______________________
24. urin/o ______________________

Suffixes

Give the definitions of the following suffixes.

1. -al ______________________
2. -ar ______________________
3. -cele ______________________
4. -dynia ______________________
5. -y ______________________
6. -ous ______________________
7. -ectomy ______________________
8. -emia ______________________
9. -gram ______________________
10. -ic ______________________
11. -in ______________________
12. -ion ______________________
13. -ist ______________________
14. -itis ______________________
15. -lith ______________________
16. -logy ______________________
17. -lysis ______________________
18. -tripsy ______________________
19. -ure ______________________
20. -meter ______________________
21. -oma ______________________
22. -osis ______________________
23. -pathy ______________________
24. -plasty ______________________
25. -scope ______________________
26. -esis ______________________
27. -stomy ______________________
28. -tomy ______________________
29. -uria ______________________

Identifying Medical Terms

In the spaces provided, write the medical terms for the following meanings.

1. ______________________ Pertaining to a medication that decreases urine production and secretion
2. ______________________ Surgical excision of the bladder or part of the bladder
3. ______________________ Inflammation of the bladder
4. ______________________ Difficult or painful urination
5. ______________________ Inflammation of the renal glomeruli
6. ______________________ Excessive amount of calcium in the urine
7. ______________________ Process of voiding urine
8. ______________________ Kidney stones

9. ______________________________ Pertaining to around the urethra

10. ______________________________ Pus in the urine

11. ______________________________ Surgical repair of the ureter

12. ______________________________ Analysis of urine

13. ______________________________ Physician who specializes in the study of the urinary system

Matching

Select the appropriate lettered meaning for each of the following words.

__________ **1.** ESWL

__________ **2.** hemodialysis

__________ **3.** lithotripsy

__________ **4.** peritoneal dialysis

__________ **5.** renal colic

__________ **6.** urethral stricture

__________ **7.** urgency

__________ **8.** urination

__________ **9.** urochrome

__________ **10.** urinometer

a. Sharp, severe pain in the lower back over the kidney radiating forward into the groin caused by a stone in a ureter

b. Crushing of a kidney stone

c. Process of voiding urine

d. Medical device used to crush kidney stones

e. Use of an artificial kidney to separate waste from the blood

f. Separation of waste from the blood by using a peritoneal catheter and dialysis

g. Narrowing or constriction of the urethra

h. Pigment that gives urine its normal yellow color

i. Medical instrument used to measure the specific gravity of urine

j. Sudden need to void, urinate

k. Analysis of urine

Medical Case Snapshots

This learning activity provides an opportunity to relate the medical terminology you are learning to a precise patient case presentation. In the spaces provided, write in your answers.

Case 1

A 10-year-old girl is referred to an urologist. She complained that "It hurts me every time I have to go to the bathroom and I go a lot at night." The medical term ______________ (means painful urination) and the term ______________ (means urination during the night). The clean-catch urine specimen appeared smoky and had an unpleasant odor. Under microscopic examination, the urine was found to contain red blood cells. This condition is called ______________.

Case 2

The physician ordered a complete UA, an abbreviation for ________________. The results show: *color* (reddish), which indicated the presence of ______________; *reaction* 9.0 pH (alkaline urine), which is indicative of ______________ ______________ ______________; and *nitrites positive*, indicating ________________ (presence of bacteria in the urine). The diagnosis of ______________ (inflammation of the bladder) was confirmed.

Case 3

A 30-year-old male is seen in the ER. He complains of sharp, severe pain in the lower back, over the kidney, radiating forward into his groin. Because of the patient's symptoms, the physician wants to evaluate him for ______________ (commonly called kidney stones). Two treatment techniques that can be used are: ESWL, which stands for ______________ ______________ ______________ lithotripsy, and PUL, or percutaneous ______________ lithotripsy. See Figures 12.8 and 12.15.

Study and Review III

Building Medical Terms

Using the following word parts, fill in the blanks to build the correct medical terms.

olig-	meat/o	-ion
cyst/o	nephr/o	-uria
continence	ren	

Definition	Medical Term
1. Indicates the presence of serum protein in the urine	albumin______
2. X-ray record of the bladder	________gram
3. Inability to hold or control urination or defecation	in__________
4. Incision of the urinary meatus to enlarge the opening	________tomy
5. Process of urination	micturit______
6. Kidney stones	_______lithiasis

Definition	Medical Term
7. Scanty, decreased amount of urine	________uria
8. Literally means excessive secretion and discharge of urine	poly________
9. Pertaining to the kidney	__________al
10. Process of voiding urine	urinat_______

Combining Form Challenge

Using the combining forms provided, write the medical term correctly.

cyst/o	lith/o	noct/o
glycos/o	nephr/o	ureter/o

1. Hernia of the bladder that protrudes into the vagina: __________ cele

2. Presence of glucose in the urine: __________ uria

3. Crushing of a kidney stone: __________ tripsy

4. Kidney tumor: __________ oma

5. Urination during the night: __________ uria

6. Disease of the ureter: __________ pathy

Select the Right Term

Select the correct answer, and write it on the line provided.

1. Presence of calcium in the urine.

anuria **calciuria** **calculus** **calcuria**

2. Pathological condition in which the body tissues contain an accumulation of fluid is __________.

excretory **diuresis** **enuresis** **edema**

3. Presence of red blood cells in the urine is __________.

glycosuria **hematuria** **calciuria** **ketonuria**

4. Condition of hardening of the kidney is ________.

nephology **nephrectomy** **nephritis** **nephrosclerosis**

5. Inflammation of the kidney and renal pelvis is __________.

pyelitis **pyelolithotomy** **pyelonephritis** **pyelcystitis**

6. Sharp, severe pain in the lower back over the kidney is __________.

renal failure **renal colic** **rennin** **stricture**

Diagnostic and Laboratory Tests

Select the best answer to each multiple-choice question. Circle the letter of your choice.

1. Urine test to determine the glomerular filtration rate.
   - **a.** BUN
   - **b.** creatinine
   - **c.** creatinine clearance
   - **d.** KUB

2. Urine test to determine the presence of microorganisms.
   - **a.** BUN
   - **b.** creatinine
   - **c.** urine culture
   - **d.** KUB

3. Test to visualize the kidneys, ureters, and bladder. A radiopaque substance is used and x-rays are taken.
   - **a.** cystoscopy
   - **b.** intravenous pyelography
   - **c.** KUB
   - **d.** renal biopsy

4. Use of high-frequency sound waves to visualize the kidneys.
   - **a.** retrograde pyelography
   - **b.** intravenous pyelography
   - **c.** ultrasonography
   - **d.** cystoscopy

5. Flat-plate x-ray of the abdomen to indicate the size and position of the kidneys, ureters, and bladder.
   - **a.** cystoscopy
   - **b.** KUB
   - **c.** BUN
   - **d.** retrograde pyelography

Abbreviations

Place the correct word, phrase, or abbreviation in the space provided.

1. acute glomerulonephritis ______________________________
2. BUN ______________________________
3. chronic kidney disease ______________________________
4. cysto ______________________________
5. GU ______________________________
6. HD ______________________________
7. intravenous pyelogram ______________________________
8. PD ______________________________
9. pH ______________________________
10. urinalysis ______________________________

Practical Application

Medical Record Analysis

This exercise contains information, abbreviations, and medical terminology from an actual medical record or case study that has been adapted for this text. The names and any personal information are made up by the author. Read and study each form or case study and then answer the questions that follow. You may refer to Appendix III, *Abbreviations and Symbols*.

Note: Congress passed the Clinical Laboratory Improvement Amendments (CLIA) in 1988, establishing quality standards for all laboratory testing to ensure the accuracy, reliability, and timeliness of patient test results regardless of where the test was performed.

FLOYD PRIMARY CARE

Task Edit View Time Scale Options Help Date: 23 May 2017

Smith-Jones Lab
35 Sinclair Avenue
Rome, GA 30165
(123) 456-7890
CLIA: 12Do840311

Lab Director: Sandra Marie Smith, MD

Patient ID: 184234
Patient Name: Reynolds, Charles L.
Date of Birth: 02/20/40
Age: 77 years
Gender: M

Draw Date: 05/19/17
Draw Time: 10:49 AM
Accession #: 71189

Ordering Dr: Smith, Sandra M.

Urinalysis	Result	Reference	Lo	Hi
Color	Yellow	Yellow to amber		
Appearance	Clear	Clear		
Specific Gravity (sp. gr.)	1.010	1.001–1.035		
pH	7.0	4.6 to 8.0		
Protein	Negative	Negative		
Glucose	Negative	Negative		
Ketones	Negative	Negative		
Bilirubin	Negative	Negative		
Blood	Negative	Negative		
Nitrites	Negative	Negative		
Urobilinogen	0.4	0.1 to 1.0		

Action: Patient to be notified of results **Reviewed by:** SJR **Date:** 05/23/17

Medical Record Questions

Place the correct answer in the space provided.

1. What is the normal color of urine? ____________________
2. Define specific gravity and give the normal sp. gr. of urine. ____________________
3. This patient's pH was 7.0. Is this higher or lower than the average pH? ____________________
4. This patient's report indicated a urobilinogen of 0.4. Is this within normal range? ____________________
5. What would an increased amount of urobilinogen indicate? ____________________

MyMedicalTerminologyLab™

MyMedicalTerminologyLab is a premium online homework management system that includes a host of features to help you study. Registered users will find:

- A multitude of quizzes and activities built within the MyLab platform
- Powerful tools that track and analyze your results—allowing you to create a personalized learning experience
- Videos and audio pronunciations to help enrich your progress
- Streaming lesson presentations (Guided Lectures) and self-paced learning modules
- A space where you and your instructor can check your progress and manage your assignments

Study and Review I

Anatomy and Physiology

Write your answers to the following questions.

1. Name the primary glands of the endocrine system.

   a. ______________________ b. ______________________

   c. ______________________ d. ______________________

   e. ______________________ f. ______________________

   g. ______________________ h. ______________________

2. State the vital function of the endocrine system. ______________________

   ____

3. Define hormone. ______________________

4. State the vital role of the hypothalamus in regulating endocrine functions. ______________________

   ____

   ____

   ____

5. Why is the pituitary gland known as the master gland of the body? ______________________

   ____

6. Name the hormones secreted by the anterior lobe (*adenohypophysis*) of the pituitary gland.

   a. ______________________ b. ______________________

   c. ______________________ d. ______________________

   e. ______________________ f. ______________________

   g. ______________________

7. Name the hormones secreted by the posterior lobe (*neurohypophysis*) of the pituitary gland.

   a. ______________________ b. ______________________

8. The pineal gland secretes the hormones ______________________ and ______________________.

9. State the vital role of the thyroid gland. ______________________

10. Name the hormones stored and secreted by the thyroid gland.

a. ______________________ **b.** ______________________

c. ______________________

11. Parathyroid hormone (*parathormone*) is essential for the maintenance of a normal level of ______________________ and also plays a role in the metabolism of ______________________.

12. Insulin is essential for the maintenance of a normal level of ______________________.

13. The adrenal cortex secretes a group of hormones known as the ______________________, the ______________________, and the ______________________.

14. Name four functions of cortisol.

a. ______________________ **b.** ______________________

c. ______________________ **d.** ______________________

15. Name four functions of corticosterone.

a. ______________________ **b.** ______________________

c. ______________________ **d.** ______________________

16. ______________________ is the principal mineralocorticoid secreted by the adrenal cortex.

17. Define androgen. ______________________

18. Name the three main catecholamines synthesized, secreted, and stored by the adrenal medulla.

a. ______________________ **b.** ______________________

c. ______________________

19. Name three functions of the hormone epinephrine.

a. ______________________

b. ______________________

c. ______________________

20. The ovaries produce the hormones ______________________ and ______________________.

21. The testes produce the hormone ______________________.

22. Name the two hormones secreted by the thymus.

a. ______________________ **b.** ______________________

23. Name the four hormones secreted by the gastrointestinal mucosa.

a. ______________________ **b.** ______________________

c. ______________________ **d.** ______________________

ANATOMY LABELING

Identify the structures shown below by filling in the blanks.

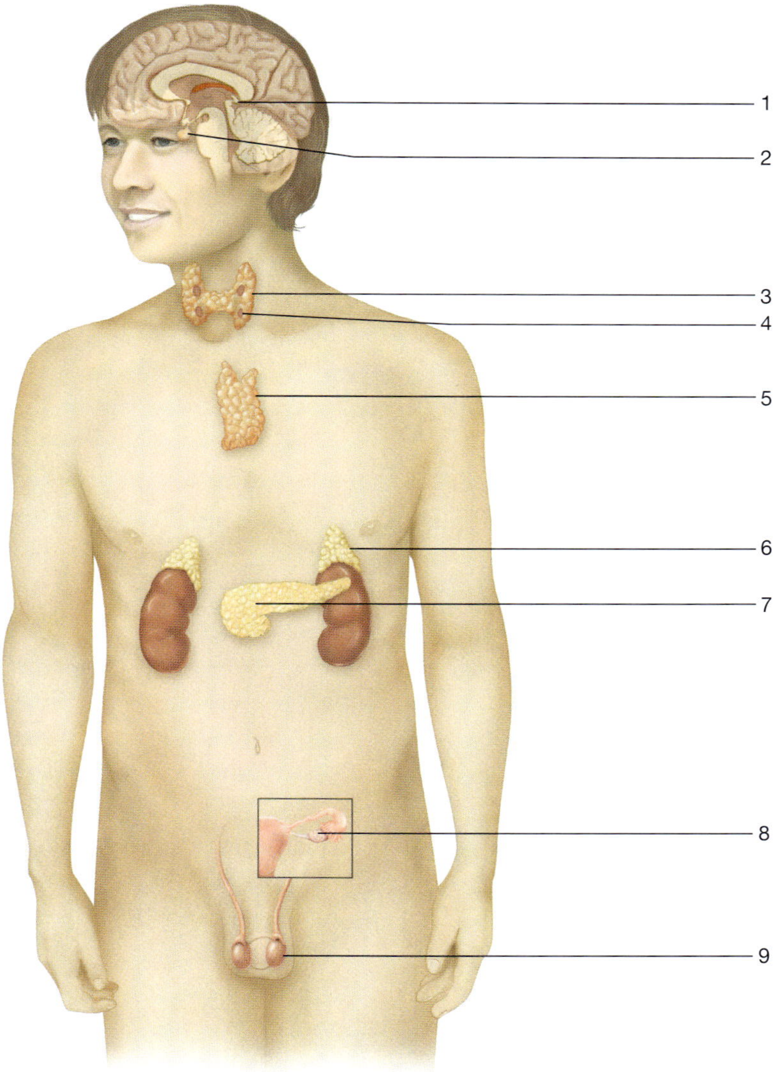

Study and Review II

Word Parts

Prefixes

Give the definitions of the following prefixes.

1. dia- ______________________
2. endo- ______________________
3. eu- ______________________
4. ex- ______________________
5. exo- ______________________
6. hyper- ______________________
7. hypo- ______________________
8. para- ______________________
9. pro- ______________________
10. epi- ______________________

Combining Forms

Give the definitions of the following combining forms.

1. acid/o ______________________
2. acr/o ______________________
3. aden/o ______________________
4. adren/o ______________________
5. andr/o ______________________
6. cortic/o ______________________
7. crin/o ______________________
8. estr/o ______________________
9. ger/o ______________________
10. gigant/o ______________________
11. gluc/o ______________________
12. gonad/o ______________________
13. hirsut/o ______________________
14. insulin/o ______________________
15. kal/i ______________________
16. myx/o ______________________
17. pancreat/o ______________________
18. test/o ______________________
19. thym/o ______________________
20. thyr/o ______________________
21. toxic/o ______________________
22. viril/o ______________________

Suffixes

Give the definitions of the following suffixes.

1. -al ______________________
2. -gen ______________________
3. -ar ______________________
4. -betes ______________________
5. -ectomy ______________________
6. -edema ______________________
7. -emia ______________________
8. -genic ______________________
9. -ia ______________________
10. -ic ______________________
11. -ism ______________________
12. -ist ______________________
13. -itis ______________________
14. -logy ______________________
15. -one ______________________
16. -megaly ______________________
17. -oid ______________________
18. -oma ______________________
19. -osis ______________________
20. -pathy ______________________
21. -ine ______________________
22. -physis ______________________
23. -in ______________________
24. -y ______________________

Identifying Medical Terms

In the spaces provided, write the medical terms for the following meanings.

1. ______________________ Tumor of a gland
2. ______________________ Congenital deficiency in secretion of the thyroid hormones characterized by arrested physical and mental development
3. ______________________ General term used to describe diseases characterized by excessive discharge of urine
4. ______________________ Study of the endocrine system
5. ______________________ Normal activity of the thyroid gland
6. ______________________ Pertains to a type of gland that secretes into ducts (duct glands)
7. ______________________ Pathological condition of being abnormally large
8. ______________________ General classification of the adrenal cortex hormones
9. ______________________ Condition of excessive amounts of potassium in the blood

10. ______________________________ Condition caused by deficient internal secretion of the gonads

11. ______________________________ Pertaining to drowsiness; sluggishness

12. ______________________________ Inflammation of the thymus

Matching

Select the appropriate lettered meaning for each of the following words.

___________ **1.** aldosterone
___________ **2.** androgen
___________ **3.** progesterone
___________ **4.** cortisone
___________ **5.** dopamine
___________ **6.** epinephrine
___________ **7.** insulin
___________ **8.** iodine
___________ **9.** thyroxine
___________ **10.** vasopressin

a. Also called *antidiuretic hormone*, *ADH*
b. Hormone released during the second half of the menstrual cycle
c. Acts to regulate the metabolism of glucose
d. Hormone produced by the thyroid gland
e. Essential in regulating electrolyte and water balance by promoting sodium and chloride reabsorption and potassium excretion
f. Hormones that produce or stimulate the development of male characteristics
g. Glucocorticoid (steroid) hormone used as an anti-inflammatory agent
h. Intermediate substance in the synthesis of norepinephrine
i. Also called *adrenaline*
j. Trace mineral that aids in the development and functioning of the thyroid gland
k. Hormone produced by the testes

MEDICAL CASE SNAPSHOTS

This learning activity provides an opportunity to relate the medical terminology you are learning to a precise patient case presentation. In the spaces provided, write in your answers.

Case 1

A 54-year-old female presents with fatigue, muscular weakness, and a round, red face. These are symptoms associated with _______________ (disease that results from the hypersecretion of cortisol). Prolonged administration of large doses of ACTH can also cause this condition. Two characteristic signs of this condition are: a _______________ _______________ and a moon face.

Case 2

A 15-year-old male complains of being "thirsty, hungry, and frequent urination." The medical terms for his complaints are: ________________ or excessive thirst, ________________ or extreme hunger, and ________________ or frequent urination.

Case 3

The patient is a 48-year-old female presenting with marked protrusion of the eyeballs indicative of ________________ goiter, sometimes called ________________ disease. People with this condition develop eye problems including bulging, red, or ________________ eyes, sensitivity to ________________, and ________________ or double vision.

Study and Review III

Building Medical Terms

Using the following word parts, fill in the blanks to build the correct medical terms.

hypo-	letharg	-in
adren	-one	-edema
dwarf	-ism	-al

Definition	Medical Term
1. Pertaining to the adrenal glands; also called suprarenal glands	___________al
2. Glucocorticoid hormone secreted by the adrenal cortex	cortis________
3. Condition of being abnormally small	___________ism
4. Pathological condition of being abnormally large	gigant________
5. Abnormal condition characterized by excessive growth of hair	hirsut________
6. Literally means *any undergrowth*; also called the pituitary gland	________physis
7. Hormone produced by the beta cells of the islets of Langerhans	insul_________
8. Pertaining to drowsiness, sluggish	___________ic
9. Literally means *condition of mucus swelling*	myx_________
10. Endocrine gland shaped like a small pine cone	pine_________

Combining Form Challenge

Using the combining forms provided, write the medical term correctly.

aden/o	estr/o	thym/o
andr/o	insulin/o	thyr/o

1. Any disease condition of a gland: _______osis

2. Hormone that produces the development of male characteristics: _______gen

3. Female sex hormone produced in the ovaries: ______gen

4. Formation or production of insulin: _______genic

5. Surgical excision of the thymus gland: _______ectomy

6. Endocrine gland located in the neck: _______oid

Select the Right Term

Select the correct answer, and write it on the line provided.

1. Characterized (in the adult) by marked enlargement and elongation of the bones of the face, jaw, and extremities is __________.

   Addison disease **acidosis** **acromegaly** **adenoma**

2. General term used to describe diseases characterized by excessive discharge of urine is __________.

   diabetes **cretinism** **Cushing** **exophthalmic**

3. Hormone produced by the adrenal medulla, also called adrenaline, is __________.

   dopamine **epinephrine** **estrogen** **norepinephrine**

4. Pathological condition in which the thyroid gland produces inadequate amounts of thyroid hormone is __________.

   hyperthyroidism **hypophysis** **hypothyroidism** **hypogonadism**

5. Pathological condition of premature old age occurring in childhood is __________.

   myxedema **lethargic** **pituitarism** **progeria**

6. Pathological condition in which secondary male characteristics are produced in a female is __________.

   thyrotoxicosis **progeria** **hypoparathyroidism** **virilism**

Diagnostic and Laboratory Tests

Select the best answer to each multiple-choice question. Circle the letter of your choice.

1. A test performed on urine to determine the amount of epinephrine and norepinephrine present.
   a. catecholamines
   b. corticotropin
   c. protein-bound iodine
   d. total calcium

2. Increased levels can indicate prediabetes or diabetes mellitus.
   a. protein-bound iodine
   b. total calcium
   c. fasting blood sugar
   d. thyroid scan

3. Test used to detect tumors of the thyroid gland.
   a. thyroxine
   b. total calcium
   c. thyroid scan
   d. protein-bound iodine

4. Blood sugar test performed at specific intervals after the patient has been given a certain amount of glucose.
   a. fasting blood sugar
   b. glucose tolerance test
   c. protein-bound iodine
   d. corticotropin

5. A test used in the diagnosing of adrenal tumors.
   a. 17-HCS
   b. 17-OHCS
   c. 17-KS
   d. 17-HDL

Abbreviations

Place the correct word, phrase, or abbreviation in the space provided.

1. basal metabolic rate ____________
2. diabetes mellitus ____________
3. FBS ____________
4. GTT ____________
5. protein-bound iodine ____________
6. PTH ____________
7. RIA ____________
8. somatotropin hormone ____________
9. TSH ____________
10. VP ____________

Practical Application

Case Study Analysis

This exercise contains information, abbreviations, and medical terminology from an actual medical record or case study that has been adapted for this text. The names and any personal information have been created by the author. Read and study each form or case study and then answer the questions that follow. You may refer to Appendix III, *Abbreviations and Symbols*.

DIABETES CASE STUDY

Task | Edit | View | Time Scale | Options | Help — Date: 17 May 2017

Meet Matthew J. Marshall

Matthew is a 15 y/o white male c/o being "thirsty, hungry, and urinating a lot." He states, "I am tired and just don't have any energy. I eat like a horse, but I stay hungry. I am afraid that I have 'sugar.' My dad and my grandfather both take insulin."

Signs and Symptoms: Polydipsia, polyphagia, polyuria, and fatigue.
Family history is notable for type 1 diabetes in father and paternal grandfather; his maternal grandmother has heart disease. **Allergies:** NKDA. Typically, for a patient with this complaint and history, type 2 diabetes would be considered.

The pertinent findings on physical exam:

Vital Signs: T: 98.4 F; P: 78; R: 18; BP: 132/70

Ht: 5′ 5″

Wt: 160 lb

General Appearance: Overweight for age. BMI: 26.6

Heart: Regular rate and rhythm. No murmurs. Lungs: CTA. Abd: Noted excessive adipose tissue. Soft, nontender, no masses, no liver enlargement. Skin: Warm and dry, no lesions, no discoloration of lower extremities.

The Plan for Diagnosis and Treatment:

1. Send to lab for Hb A1C and schedule FBS, ASAP.
2. Recommend that Matthew attend the next health education seminar. One or both parents are to attend the seminar with him. Explain that individuals who are overweight, have a BMI greater than or equal to 25, and who have immediate family members with diabetes are at a higher risk of developing diabetes. Note: For more information on diabetes, call (800) DIABETES.
3. Patient is to return in 1 week for test results. If indicated, proper medication regimen will be initiated for Matthew.

Case Study Questions

Place the correct answer in the space provided

1. Why is Matthew concerned that he may have "sugar"? ______________________

2. To rule out diabetes mellitus, the physician ordered a ______________________ test and a ______________________ ASAP.

3. What are the three classic symptoms of diabetes mellitus that Matthew stated?
______________________ ______________________ ______________________

4. What does the abbreviation *FBS* mean? ______________________

5. A BMI over ______________________ may indicate a higher risk of developing diabetes.

Study and Review I

Anatomy and Physiology

Write your answers to the following questions.

1. Name the two interconnected divisions of the nervous system.

a. ______________________ **b.** ______________________

2. ______________________ are the structural and functional units of the nervous system.

3. Describe an axon. ______________________

4. Describe a dendrite. ______________________

5. State an action of sensory neurons. ______________________

6. Define the following terms:

a. Nerve fiber ______________________

b. Nerve ______________________

c. Tracts ______________________

7. The central nervous system consists of the ______________________ and the ______________________.

8. Name the three meninges enclosing the brain.

a. ______________________ **b.** ______________________

c. ______________________

9. Name four major structures of the brain.

   a. ______________________________ b. ______________________________

   c. ______________________________ d. ______________________________

10. The ______________________________ has been identified as the brain's major motor area.

11. The parietal lobe is also known as the ______________________________

12. The temporal lobe contains centers for ______________________________ and ______________________________ input.

13. The occipital lobe is the primary area for ______________________________.

14. State the functions of the thalamus.

   a. ______________________________ b. ______________________________

15. State three functions of the hypothalamus.

   a. ______________________________ b. ______________________________

   c. ______________________________

16. The cerebellum plays an important role in the integration of ______________________________ and ______________________________.

17. State five functions of the medulla oblongata.

   a. ______________________________ b. ______________________________

   c. ______________________________ d. ______________________________

   e. ______________________________

18. State the three functions of the spinal cord.

   a. ______________________________ b. ______________________________

   c. ______________________________

19. The normal adult has between ______________________________ and ______________________________ mL of cerebrospinal fluid in circulation.

20. State four functions of the autonomic nervous system.

a. ______________________ **b.** ______________________

c. ______________________ **d.** ______________________

21. Name the two divisions of the autonomic nervous system.

a. ______________________ **b.** ______________________

ANATOMY LABELING

Identify the structures shown below by filling in the blanks.

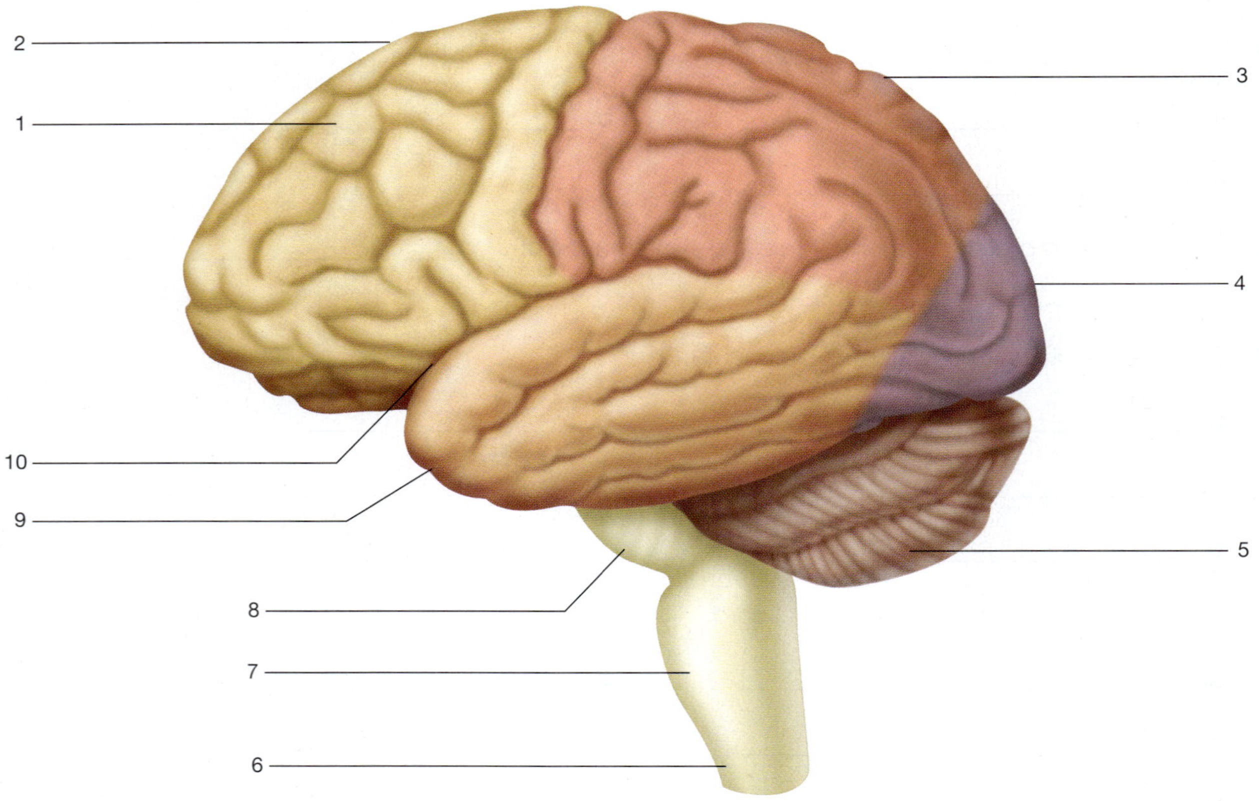

Study and Review II

Word Parts

Prefixes

Give the definitions of the following prefixes.

1. a- ______________________
2. an- ______________________
3. astro- ______________________
4. brady- ______________________
5. de- ______________________
6. dys- ______________________
7. epi- ______________________
8. hemi- ______________________
9. hydro- ______________________
10. hyper- ______________________
11. intra- ______________________
12. micro- ______________________
13. oligo- ______________________
14. par- ______________________
15. para- ______________________
16. poly- ______________________
17. quadri- ______________________
18. sub- ______________________

Combining Forms

Give the definitions of the following combining forms.

1. cephal/o ______________________
2. cerebell/o ______________________
3. cerebr/o ______________________
4. crani/o ______________________
5. dendr/o ______________________
6. disk/o ______________________
7. dur/o ______________________
8. electr/o ______________________
9. encephal/o ______________________
10. esthesi/o ______________________
11. hypn/o ______________________
12. lamin/o ______________________
13. mening/o ______________________
14. myel/o ______________________
15. narc/o ______________________
16. neur/o ______________________
17. pallid/o ______________________
18. poli/o ______________________
19. somn/o ______________________
20. spin/o ______________________

21. spondyl/o ____________________ **22.** vag/o ____________________

23. ventricul/o ____________________

Suffixes

Give the definitions of the following suffixes.

1. -al ____________________ **2.** -algesia ____________________

3. -algia ____________________ **4.** -ar ____________________

5. -asthenia ____________________ **6.** -blast ____________________

7. -cele ____________________ **8.** -cyte ____________________

9. -desis ____________________ **10.** -ectomy ____________________

11. -edema ____________________ **12.** -esthesia ____________________

13. -glia ____________________ **14.** -gram ____________________

15. -graphy ____________________ **16.** -ia ____________________

17. -ic ____________________ **18.** -ion ____________________

19. -ism ____________________ **20.** -ist ____________________

21. -itis ____________________ **22.** -kinesia ____________________

23. -kinesis ____________________ **24.** -lepsy ____________________

25. -lexia ____________________ **26.** -logy ____________________

27. -troph(y) ____________________ **28.** -scopy ____________________

29. -oma ____________________ **30.** -osis ____________________

31. -paresis ____________________ **32.** -pathy ____________________

33. -phagia ____________________ **34.** -phasia ____________________

35. -praxia ____________________ **36.** -sthenia ____________________

37. -taxia ____________________ **38.** -tomy ____________________

39. -us ____________________ **40.** -y ____________________

Identifying Medical Terms

In the spaces provided, write the medical terms for the following meanings.

1. ______________________ Condition in which there is a loss or lack of memory
2. ______________________ Condition in which there is a lack of the sensation of pain
3. ______________________ Loss or lack of the ability to eat or swallow
4. ______________________ Neurological sign and symptom consisting of lack of coordination of muscle movements
5. ______________________ Head pain; headache
6. ______________________ Pertaining to the cerebellum
7. ______________________ Surgical excision of a portion of the skull
8. ______________________ Condition in which an individual has difficulty reading and writing words even though vision and intelligence are unimpaired
9. ______________________ Inflammation of the brain
10. ______________________ Literally means pertaining to situated on the dura mater
11. ______________________ Slight paralysis that affects one side of the body
12. ______________________ Inflammation of the meninges of the spinal cord or brain
13. ______________________ Pain in a nerve or nerves
14. ______________________ Inflammation of a nerve
15. ______________________ Nerve cell, neuron
16. ______________________ The study of the nervous system
17. ______________________ Tumor of nerve cells and nerve fibers
18. ______________________ Pathological loss of sensation or an impairment of motor function
19. ______________________ Literally means *inflammation involving many nerves*
20. ______________________ Condition of sleepwalking
21. ______________________ Surgical incision of the vagus nerve
22. ______________________ X-ray of the cerebral ventricles

Matching

Select the appropriate lettered meaning for each of the following words.

_________ **1.** acetylcholine
_________ **2.** Alzheimer disease
_________ **3.** stroke
_________ **4.** endorphins
_________ **5.** epilepsy
_________ **6.** palsy
_________ **7.** diskectomy
_________ **8.** epiduroscopy
_________ **9.** dementia
_________ **10.** sciatica

a. Group of symptoms marked by memory loss and other cognitive functions

b. Chemical substances produced in the brain that act as natural analgesics (*opiates*) and provide feelings of pleasure

c. Cerebrovascular accident

d. The most common cause of dementia among older adults

e. A neurological disorder involving repeated seizures of any type

f. Used for back pain relief when all other conservative treatments have failed

g. Cholinergic neurotransmitter

h. Pathological loss of sensation or an impairment of motor function

i. Severe pain along the course of the sciatic nerve

j. Surgical excision of an intervertebral disk

k. Anxiety syndrome and panic disorder

Medical Case Snapshots

This learning activity provides an opportunity to relate the medical terminology you are learning to a precise patient case presentation. In the spaces provided, write in your answers.

Case 1

An 8-year-old girl was accompanied by her mother to the doctor's office. The mother states that, about 2 years ago, her daughter was diagnosed with _________ (which is a neurological disorder involving repeated seizures). The majority of diagnosed cases of this disorder are ___________ as their causes cannot be identified.

Case 2

The 74-year-old male was seen by his physician. He was in acute pain and complaining of severe itching around his waistline. Examination of his torso revealed evidence of a viral disease characterized by painful vesicular eruptions. This disease, known as _________ _________ is caused by the varicella-zoster virus, the same virus that causes _________. The common name for this condition is _________.

Case 3

A 70-year-old male diagnosed with Parkinson disease was seen by a neurologist. The patient had moderate to severe tremor (worse in the left hand than the right), difficulty in movement with _________ or abnormal slowness of motion, with freezing in place or _____________. The physician discussed with the patient and his wife the possibility of a surgical procedure known as a _________________ wherein there is destruction of the globus pallidus of the brain.

Study and Review III

Building Medical Terms

Using the following word parts, fill in the blanks to build the correct medical terms.

an-	papill	-esthesia
quadri-	-kinesia	-tomy
concuss	-itis	
neur	-ectomy	

Definition	Medical Term
1. Condition in which there is a lack of the sensation of pain	_______algesia
2. Abnormal slowness of movement	brady ________
3. Head injury with a transient loss of brain function	__________ion
4. Inflammation of the brain	encephal _____
5. Surgical excision of a vertebral posterior arch	lamin ________
6. Pain in a nerve or nerves	_________algia
7. Swelling of the optic disk, usually caused by ICP	_______edema
8. Abnormal sensation, feeling of numbness, or prickling	par _________
9. Paralysis of all four extremities and usually the trunk	________plegia
10. Surgical incision of the vagus nerve	vago ________

Combining Form Challenge

Using the combining forms provided, write the medical term correctly.

cephal/o	encephal/o	mening/o
cran/i	hypn/o	neur/o

1. Head pain; headache: ________algia

2. Surgical excision of a portion of the skull: ________ectomy

3. Any pathological dysfunction of the brain: ________pathy

4. Artificially induced trancelike state resembling sleepwalking: ________osis

5. Inflammation of the meninges of the spinal cord or brain: ________itis

6. Supporting or connective tissue cells of the central nervous system: ________glia

Select the Right Term

Select the correct answer, and write it on the line provided.

1. Inability to remain still; motor restlessness and anxiety is ____________.

   akathisia **akinesia** **aphagia** **apraxia**

2. Literally means *loss or lack of the sense of feeling* is ____________.

   analgesia **anesthesia** **aphasia** **asthenia**

3. Unconscious state or stupor from which the patient cannot be aroused is ____________.

   chorea **concussion** **coma** **epilepsy**

4. Group of symptoms marked by memory loss and other cognitive functions is ____________.

   dyslexia **dysphasia** **hypnosis** **dementia**

5. Increased muscular movement and motion is ____________.

   hyperesthesia **narcolepsy** **hyperkinesis** **paresis**

6. Death of focal brain tissue that occurs when the brain does not get sufficient blood and oxygen is ____________.

   sundowning **stroke** **syncope** **palsy**

Diagnostic and Laboratory Tests

Select the best answer to each multiple-choice question. Circle the letter of your choice.

1. Diagnostic procedure used to study the structure of the brain.
   - **a.** computed tomography
   - **b.** echoencephalography
   - **c.** electroencephalography
   - **d.** myelogram
2. Process of using ultrasound to determine the presence of a centrally located mass in the brain.
   - **a.** computed tomography
   - **b.** echoencephalography
   - **c.** electroencephalography
   - **d.** myelogram
3. X-ray of the spinal canal after the injection of a radiopaque dye.
   - **a.** cerebral angiography
   - **b.** computed tomography
   - **c.** myelogram
   - **d.** ultrasonography
4. Computer-based nuclear imaging procedure that can produce three-dimensional pictures of actual organ functioning.
   - **a.** electroencephalography
   - **b.** myelogram
   - **c.** ultrasonography
   - **d.** positron emission tomography
5. Use of high-frequency sound waves to produce an image on a computer screen.
   - **a.** electroencephalography
   - **b.** myelogram
   - **c.** ultrasonography
   - **d.** positron emission tomography

Abbreviations

Place the correct word, phrase, or abbreviation in the space provided.

1. Alzheimer disease ____________________
2. amyotrophic lateral sclerosis ____________________
3. CNS ____________________
4. CP ____________________
5. computed tomography ____________________
6. herniated disk syndrome ____________________
7. ICP ____________________
8. LP ____________________
9. MS ____________________
10. positron emission tomography ____________________

Practical Application

Medical Record Analysis

This exercise contains information, abbreviations, and medical terminology from an actual medical record or case study that has been adapted for this text. The names and any personal information have been created by the author. Read and study each form or case study and then answer the questions that follow. You may refer to Appendix III, *Abbreviations and Symbols*.

OXFORD NEUROLOGICAL CENTER

Task Edit View Time Scale Options Help Date: 17 May 2017

7894 Hazelbrook Drive
Centreville, VA 30120
(123) 456-7890

Marcus James Madison, MD Charles Robert Jones, MD Nagoya T. Yung, MD

Summary Report

Patient: Brown, James E. **Age:** 78 **Gender:** Male **Date:** 05/10/17

James E. Brown, age 78, has advanced Parkinson disease, present for 7 years. It is affecting his activities of daily living (ADL). He has difficulty bathing, dressing, and has frequent falls. He has marked hesitancy on changing directions and unsteadiness with fatigue. He can brush his teeth and wash his face.

On neurological examination he did have mild to moderate impairment in cognition and short-term memory, although he is oriented to time, place, and person. He has a mild tremor, worse in the left arm than the right. He has rigidity in the upper extremities. He has marked difficulty in movement, with long delays in initiating movement and frequent freezing in place. He has postural instability. He has mild difficulty with articulation of speech, dysarthria. His gait is characterized by shuffling strides. He can arise from a chair with difficulty only after multiple attempts. Deep tendon reflexes are symmetrical, and toes are downgoing. Cranial nerves are unremarkable.

He has been on Sinemet 25–100 mg tid for the last 6 years. I have asked him to increase his Sinemet dose to qid. Mr. Brown is to return to our office in 3 months.

Marcus James Madison, MD

Medical Record Questions

Place the correct answer in the space provided.

1. On neurological examination Mr. Brown did have mild to moderate impairment in ________________ ________________ and short-term memory.

2. Mr. Brown has a mild ________________________________, worse in the left arm than the right.

3. What does *dysarthria* mean? ________________________________

4. Sinemet 25–100 mg is classified as a/an ________________________________ drug.

5. Why is this drug prescribed for Mr. Brown? ________________________________

Study and Review I

Anatomy and Physiology

Write your answers to the following questions.

1. The ears contain structures for both the sense of ________________ and the sense of ________________.

2. Name the three divisions of the ear.

a. ________________ **b.** ________________

c. ________________

3. The external ear consists of the ________________ and the ________________.

4. Which structure of the external ear collects sound waves? ________________

5. State the two functions of cerumen.

a. ________________ **b.** ________________

6. Name the three ossicles of the middle ear.

a. ______________________ b. ______________________

c. ______________________

7. State the function of the ossicles. ____

____

8. State two functions of the middle ear.

a. ______________________ b. ______________________

9. The bony labyrinth of the inner ear consists of the ____________________,

____________________, and the ____________________.

10. Name the three divisions of the membranous labyrinth.

a. ______________________ b. ______________________

c. ______________________

11. Located on the basilar membrane is the ____________________, containing hair cell sensory receptors for the sense of hearing.

12. The ____________________ is a bony structure located between the cochlea and the three semicircular canals.

13. The auditory nerve is also known as the ____________________.

14. Dizziness and ____________________ are associated with the continued movement of the fluid in the semicircular canals due to gravitational influences.

15. Name the two types of fluid found in the ear.

a. ______________________ b. ______________________

ANATOMY LABELING

Identify the structures shown below by filling in the blanks.

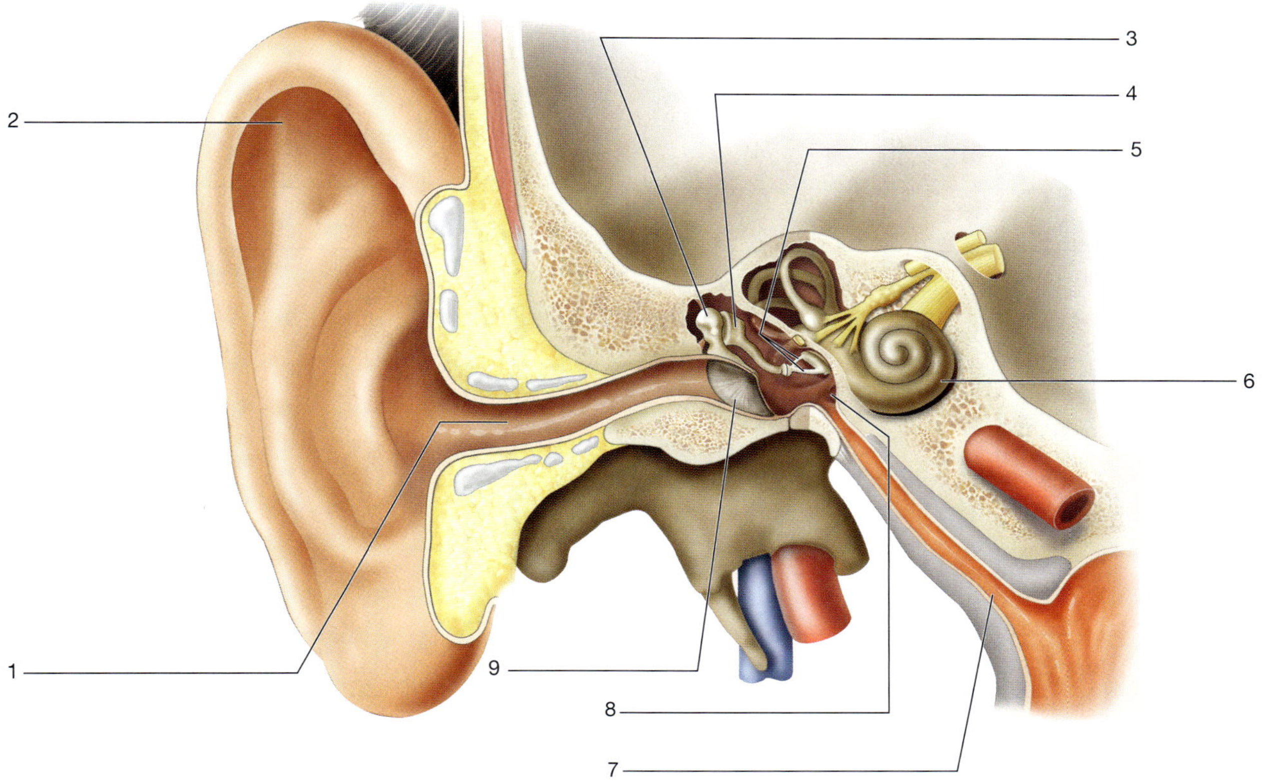

Study and Review II

Word Parts

Prefixes

Give the definitions of the following prefixes.

1. end- ____________________
2. endo- ____________________
3. peri- ____________________
4. bin- ____________________
5. mon(o)- ____________________

Combining Forms

Give the definitions of the following combining forms.

1. audi/o ____________________
2. aur/i ____________________
3. chol/e ____________________
4. cochle/o ____________________
5. electr/o ____________________
6. labyrinth/o ____________________
7. laryng/o ____________________
8. mast/o ____________________
9. myring/o ____________________
10. neur/o ____________________
11. ot/o ____________________
12. pharyng/o ____________________
13. presby/o ____________________
14. py/o ____________________
15. scler/o ____________________
16. staped/o ____________________
17. steat/o ____________________
18. tympan/o ____________________

Suffixes

Give the definitions of the following suffixes.

1. -al ____________________
2. -algia ____________________
3. -cusis ____________________
4. -ectomy ____________________
5. -gram ____________________
6. -graphy ____________________
7. -ic ____________________
8. -ist ____________________

9. -itis ______________________
10. -lith ______________________
11. -logy ______________________
12. -lymph ______________________
13. -meter ______________________
14. -metry ______________________
15. -oid ______________________
16. -oma ______________________
17. -osis ______________________
18. -plasty ______________________
19. -rrhea ______________________
20. -scope ______________________
21. -tome ______________________
22. -tomy ______________________
23. -y ______________________
24. -cle ______________________
25. -ion ______________________
26. -ia ______________________

Identifying Medical Terms

In the spaces provided, write the medical terms for the following meanings.

1. ______________________ One who specializes in diagnosing disorders of hearing
2. ______________________ Measurement of the hearing sense
3. ______________________ Pertaining to the sense of hearing
4. ______________________ Pertaining to within the ear
5. ______________________ Inflammation of the labyrinth
6. ______________________ Surgical repair of the tympanic membrane
7. ______________________ Surgical instrument used for cutting the eardrum
8. ______________________ Pain in the ear, earache
9. ______________________ Study of the ear and larynx
10. ______________________ Pertaining to the ear and pharynx
11. ______________________ Medical instrument used to examine the ear
12. ______________________ Serum fluid of the inner ear
13. ______________________ Surgical excision of the stapes of the ear
14. ______________________ Surgical excision of the tympanic membrane
15. ______________________ The sensation of ringing or roaring sounds in one or both ears

Matching

Select the appropriate lettered meaning for each of the following words.

_____________ **1.** auricle
_____________ **2.** binaural
_____________ **3.** acoustic
_____________ **4.** equilibrium
_____________ **5.** fenestration
_____________ **6.** labyrinth
_____________ **7.** myringotomy
_____________ **8.** otoplasty
_____________ **9.** tympanoplasty
_____________ **10.** vertigo

a. State of balance
b. Inner ear
c. Surgical repair of the ear
d. Surgical repair of the tympanic membrane
e. Pertaining to both ears
f. Sensation of instability, loss of equilibrium
g. Surgical operation in which a new opening is made in the labyrinth
h. External portion of the ear
i. Pertaining to the sense of hearing
j. Surgical incision of the tympanic membrane
k. Organ of hearing

Medical Case Snapshots

This learning activity provides an opportunity to relate the medical terminology you are learning to a precise patient case presentation. In the spaces provided, write in your answers.

Case 1

The mother of a 2-year-old baby states that Takeshia has been unusually fussy for 2 days and that last night "she woke me up screaming and she felt so hot." Upon examination of the left ear the physician noted a bulging of the tympanic membrane and the presence of purulent fluid in the middle ear. In the space provided, write the medical term for this condition _____________ ___________. See Figures 15.8 and 15.9.

Case 2

A 15-year-old male is seen by an otolaryngologist. He complains of ringing in the ears and is diagnosed with _____________. When questioned, he admits to listening to loud music with headphones and that he likes going to rock concerts. Excessive noise can do permanent damage to the sensory receptors of the ________ ___ ___________.

Case 3

The 15-year-old male was referred to an ______________ who specializes in diagnosing disorders of hearing. Using an ____________ (which is a medical instrument used to measure hearing), both ears were tested, one at a time. The patient was diagnosed with a partial loss of the ability to hear in the left ear. Loss of hearing is known as __________.

Study and Review III

Building Medical Terms

Using the following word parts, fill in the blanks to build the correct medical terms.

aur	staped	-lymph
myring/o	tympan/o	-itis
ot/o	-ic	

Definition	Medical Term
1. Pertaining to the sense of hearing	acoust_______
2. Pertaining to the ear	___________al
3. Clear fluid contained within the labyrinth of the ear	endo________

Definition	Medical Term
4. Surgical instrument used for cutting the eardrum	________tome
5. Inflammation of the ear	ot________
6. Surgical repair of the ear	________plasty
7. Serum fluid of the inner ear	peri________
8. Surgical excision of the stapes in the middle ear	_______ectomy
9. Pertaining to the eardrum (tympanic membrane)	tympan______
10. Surgical repair of the tympanic membrane (eardrum)	________plasty

Combining Form Challenge

Using the combining forms provided, write the medical term correctly.

audi/o	labyrinth/o	ot/o
aur/i	myring/o	presby/o

1. Medical instrument used to measure hearing: _______meter
2. External portion of the ear; known as the pinna: _______ cle
3. Surgical excision of the labyrinth: ______ ectomy
4. Surgical repair of the tympanic membrane: ________ plasty
5. Pain in the ear; earache: ______ algia
6. Impairment of hearing that occurs with aging: ________ cusis

Select the Right Term

Select the correct answer, and write it on the line provided.

1. Record of hearing by audiometry is __________.

   acoustic **audiology** **audiogram** **aural**

2. A state of balance is ____________.

   cochlea **equilibrium** **tinnitus** **eustachian**

3. Surgical operation in which a new opening is made in the labyrinth of the inner ear to restore hearing is __________.

   labyrinthotomy **myringectomy** **fenestration** **stapedectomy**

4. Largest of the three ossicles; also called the hammer is __________.

   incus **stapes** **labyrinth** **malleus**

5. The sensation of ringing or roaring sounds in one or both ears is ____________.

tinnitus **tinitus** **presbycusis** **vertigo**

6. Small, saclike structure of the labyrinth of the inner ear is ____________.

oval window **stapes** **utricle** **incus**

Diagnostic and Laboratory Tests

Select the best answer to each multiple-choice question. Circle the letter of your choice.

1. The response to auditory stimuli that can be measured independent of the patient's subjective response.
   a. auditory-evoked response
   b. electronystagmography
   c. tuning fork test
   d. otoscopy
2. Recording of eye movement in response to specific stimuli.
   a. auditory-evoked response
   b. electronystagmography
   c. tympanometry
   d. otoscopy
3. Visual examination of the external auditory canal and the tympanic membrane.
   a. tuning fork test
   b. tympanometry
   c. electronystagmography
   d. otoscopy
4. Measurement of the movement of the tympanic membrane.
   a. tuning fork tests
   b. tympanometry
   c. otoscopy
   d. electronystagmography
5. This test utilizes a tuning fork to compare bone conduction (BC) hearing with air conduction (AC).
   a. Rinne test
   b. tympanometry
   c. otoscopy
   d. electronystagmography

Abbreviations

Place the correct word, phrase, or abbreviation in the space provided.

1. air conduction ____________________
2. bone conduction ____________________
3. db, dB ____________________
4. electronystagmography ____________________
5. ENT ____________________
6. hearing distance ____________________
7. otitis media ____________________

Practical Application

Medical Record Analysis

This exercise contains information, abbreviations, and medical terminology from an actual medical record or case study that has been adapted for this text. The names and any personal information have been created by the author. Read and study each form or case study and then answer the questions that follow. You may refer to Appendix III, *Abbreviations and Symbols*.

HOLLY HILL OTOLARYNGOLOGY CLINIC

Task Edit View Time Scale Options Help Date: 17 May 2017

112 Dogwood Blvd.
Kingwood, Texas 77339
(123) 456-7890
William R. Patel, MD, King Louis Lataif, MD,
Brittany Nicole Benz, MD

May 10, 2017
Starr J. Bentley, MD
235 Maple Lane
Kingwood, Texas 77339
Re: Takeshia Chamberlain

Dear Doctor Bentley,

Thank you for your referral of Takeshia Chamberlain, age 2, seen in my office on April 25, 2017. When seen, Takeshia had a fever of 102.2° F, with noted dark circles under both eyes and appeared to be in moderate pain. Child was pulling on her left ear and upon examination left TM red, dull, and bulging diffuse light reflex with loss of landmark. Pneumatic otoscopy revealed immobile left TM. Right TM pearly gray, landmarks intact. Nasal mucosa dark red and swollen, with moderate amount of discharge. Oral mucosa erythematous with yellow-white exudates, no lesions. Uvula rises in midline with phonation. Gag reflex present. No lymphadenopathy. Neck supple. Lungs CTA and heart normal rate and rhythm. No murmurs. Skin: no rashes or lesions, warm to the touch.

A diagnosis of acute otitis media (AOM) left ear was confirmed.

I ordered acetaminophen (Tylenol) liquid, 1.6 mL (1 teaspoon) PO every 4 hours prn for pain and fever. Amoxicillin (Amoxil) suspension 40 mg per kg per day, in three divided doses, every 8 hours for 10 days for infection. Instructed the mother on the adverse reactions to penicillin and explained that she should not give the antibiotic with soft drinks or fruit juices because the acid in these products could destroy the effectiveness of the drug. Stressed the importance of the baby taking the antibiotic as ordered for the entire 10 days and around the clock, every 8 hours. Instructed the mother to bring the baby back to the clinic if symptoms do not improve in 48–72 hours. Scheduled a follow-up visit for 3 weeks.

Best regards,
William R. Patel, MD

Medical Record Questions

Place the correct answer in the space provided.

1. In Takeshia the signs and symptoms of acute otitis media included a fever of ______________________ and the child was ______________________ on her left ear.

2. The diagnosis was determined by a visual examination of the ear called pneumatic ______________________, a physical examination of the child, and the signs and symptoms presented.

3. Acetaminophen (Tylenol) is classified as a(n) ______________________ and is given to relieve ______________________ and reduce ______________________.

4. Amoxicillin (Amoxil) is a(n) ______________________ and is given for ______________________.

5. The ______________________ in soft drinks and fruit juices can destroy the effectiveness of the ______________________ drug.

Study and Review I

Anatomy and Physiology

Write your answers to the following questions.

1. The external structures of the eye are the ______________________________,
______________________________, ______________________________, ______________________________,
and the ______________________________.

2. The orbit is lined with ____________________________ ____________________________, which cushions the eyeball.

3. The optic foramen is an opening for the ______________________________
______________________________ and ______________________________
______________________________.

4. State the functions of the muscles of the eye.

a. ____

b. ____

5. Each eye has a pair of eyelids that function to protect the eyeball from ____________________________,
____, and
______________________________.

6. Describe the conjunctiva and state its function. ____________________________________
____

7. Define lacrimal apparatus. ____

8. The internal structures of the eye are the ______________________________,
______________________________, and the ______________________________
______________________________.

9. The eyeball is the organ of ______________________________.

10. The point at which nerve fibers from the retina converge to form the optic nerve is known as the
____.

11. Define accommodation. ____

12. Match the following terms and definitions by placing the correct letter on the line provided.

____________	**1.** aqueous humor	**a.** White of the eye
____________	**2.** vitreous humor	**b.** Colored membrane attached to the ciliary body
____________	**3.** iris	**c.** Watery fluid
____________	**4.** sclera	**d.** Opening in the center of the iris
____________	**5.** uvea	**e.** Jellylike material
____________	**6.** pupil	**f.** Middle layer of the eyeball
____________	**7.** retina	**g.** Transparent anterior portion of the eyeball
____________	**8.** rods and cones	**h.** Innermost layer of the eyeball
____________	**9.** lens	**i.** Photoreceptor cells
____________	**10.** cornea	**j.** Colorless crystalline body

ANATOMY LABELING

Identify the structures shown below by filling in the blanks.

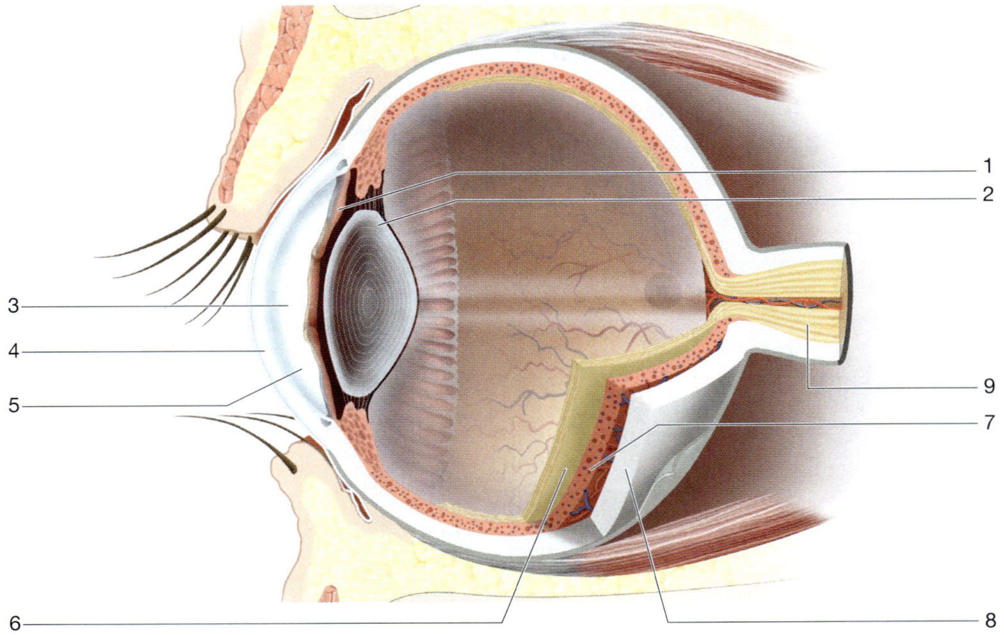

Study and Review II

Word Parts

Prefixes

Give the definitions of the following prefixes.

1. a- ____________________
2. bi- ____________________
3. en- ____________________
4. em- ____________________
5. eso- ____________________
6. hyper- ____________________
7. intra- ____________________
8. tri- ____________________
9. ex(o)- ____________________
10. hemi- ____________________
11. an- ____________________
12. retro- ____________________

Combining Forms

Give the definitions of the following combining forms.

1. ambly/o ____________________
2. anis/o ____________________
3. blephar/o ____________________
4. choroid/o ____________________
5. conjunctiv/o ____________________
6. cor/o ____________________
7. corne/o ____________________
8. cry/o ____________________
9. cycl/o ____________________
10. dacry/o ____________________
11. dipl/o ____________________
12. irid/o ____________________
13. kerat/o ____________________
14. lacrim/o ____________________
15. lent/o ____________________
16. mi/o ____________________
17. ophthalm/o ____________________
18. opt/o ____________________
19. orth/o ____________________
20. phac/o ____________________
21. phot/o ____________________
22. retin/o ____________________
23. xen/o ____________________
24. xer/o ____________________

Suffixes

Give the definitions of the following suffixes.

1. -al ______________________
2. -ar ______________________
3. -ary ______________________
4. -blast ______________________
5. -iasis ______________________
6. -ectomy ______________________
7. -gram ______________________
8. -graphy ______________________
9. -ia ______________________
10. -ic ______________________
11. -ician ______________________
12. -ion ______________________
13. -ism ______________________
14. -ist ______________________
15. -itis ______________________
16. -logy ______________________
17. -lysis ______________________
18. -plasia ______________________
19. -meter ______________________
20. -oma ______________________
21. -opia ______________________
22. -osis ______________________
23. -pathy ______________________
24. -phobia ______________________
25. -plasty ______________________
26. -plegia ______________________
27. -ptosis ______________________
28. -scope ______________________
29. -tic ______________________
30. -tomy ______________________
31. -us ______________________

Identifying Medical Terms

In the spaces provided, write the medical terms for the following meanings.

1. ______________________ Dullness of vision
2. ______________________ Pertaining to having two foci
3. ______________________ Drooping of the upper eyelid(s)
4. ______________________ Pertaining to the cornea
5. ______________________ Tumor-like swelling caused by obstruction of the tear duct(s)
6. ______________________ Double vision
7. ______________________ Normal or perfect vision
8. ______________________ Pertaining to within the eye

9. ______________________________ Inflammation of the cornea

10. ______________________________ Surgical repair of the cornea

11. ______________________________ Pertaining to tears

12. ______________________________ Pertaining to the eye

13. ______________________________ Unusual intolerance to light

Matching

Select the appropriate lettered meaning for each of the following words.

__________ **1.** anisocoria

__________ **2.** entropion

__________ **3.** cataract

__________ **4.** hemianopia

__________ **5.** phacoemulsification

__________ **6.** photocoagulation

__________ **7.** radial keratotomy

__________ **8.** retrolental fibroplasia

__________ **9.** strabismus

__________ **10.** sty(e)

a. Disorder of the eye in which the optic axes cannot be directed to the same object

b. Disease of the retinal vessels present in premature infants

c. Process of using ultrasound to disintegrate a cataract

d. Use of a laser to treat retinal detachment and/or retinal bleeding

e. Condition in which the pupils are unequal

f. Turning inward of the margin of the lower eyelid

g. Surgical procedure performed to correct myopia

h. Inability to see half of the field of vision

i. *Hordeolum*

j. Opacity of the crystalline lens or its capsule

k. Disease characterized by increased intraocular pressure

Medical Case Snapshots

This learning activity provides an opportunity to relate the medical terminology you are learning to a precise patient case presentation. In the spaces provided, write in your answers.

Case 1

A 63-year-old male presents with "trouble driving at night." He states that "bright lights hurt my eyes" and "I see halos around them." When opacity of the crystalline lens occurs in an older adult it is said to be a __________________. With this condition colors seem faded and the only effective treatment is known as __________________, a process of using ultrasound to disintegrate the lens. See Figure 16.11.

Case 2

A 17-year-old male was seen by an ophthalmologist. He complains that his eyes are really bothering him. He has been swimming every day for the past two weeks training for a swim meet. He is diagnosed with _______________ or inflammation of the conjunctiva. With this condition some of the symptoms are _______________ in the white of the eye, an increased amount of tears, a thick _______________ discharge and _______________ vision.

Case 3

A 64-year-old female is seen by her physician. Her medical history includes diagnoses of hypertension and type 2 diabetes mellitus. The results of a comprehensive eye exam revealed an increased intraocular pressure, which is known as _______________. With this condition there are no outward symptoms. Some of the predisposing factors of this condition are being over _______________ years of age, having _______________ ancestry, and diagnoses of _______________ and _______________ diabetes _______________.

Study and Review III

Building Medical Terms

Using the following word parts, fill in the blanks to build the correct medical terms.

dipl-	retin/o	-phobia
lacrim	uve	-iasis
nyctal	-ectomy	
ophthalm/o	-tic	

Definition	Medical Term
1. Double vision	_________opia
2. Surgical excision of a portion of the iris	irid___________
3. Pertains to tears	___________al
4. Pertaining to an agent that causes the pupil to contract	mio__________
5. Condition in which the individual has difficulty seeing at night	_________opia
6. Study of the eye	_________logy
7. Unusual intolerance to light	photo_______
8. Any disease of the retina	________pathy
9. Condition of in-growing eyelashes that rub against the cornea	trich__________
10. Pertaining to the second or vascular coat of the eye	___________al

Combining Form Challenge

Using the combining forms provided, write the medical term correctly.

ambly/o	cycl/o	goni/o
blephar/o	dacry/o	kerat/o

1. Dullness of vision: ___________ opia
2. Drooping of the upper eyelid(s): ___________ ptosis
3. Paralysis of the ciliary muscle: ___________ plegia
4. Tumor-like swelling caused by obstruction of the tear duct(s): ___________ oma
5. Instrument used to examine the angle of the anterior chamber of the eye: ___________ scope
6. Inflammation of the cornea: ___________ itis

Select the Right Term

Select the correct answer, and write it on the line provided.

1. Process by which the eyes make adjustments to see objects at various distances is ___________.

   amblyopia **accommodation** **anisocoria** **astigmatism**

2. Opacity of the crystalline lens or its capsule is ___________.

   cataract **chalazion** **choroiditis** **conjunctivitis**

3. Turning inward of the margin of the lower eyelid is ___________.

   enucleation **esotropia** **entropion** **exotropia**

4. Disease caused by increased intraocular pressure is ___________.

   nystagmus **hemianopia** **gonioscope** **glaucoma**

5. Vision defect in which parallel rays come to a focus beyond the retina is ___________.

   hyperopia **presbyopia** **myopia** **esotropia**

6. Inflammation of one or more of the sebaceous glands of the eyelid is ___________.

   scleritis **strabismus** **sty(e)** **xerophthalmia**

Diagnostic and Laboratory Tests

Select the best answer to each multiple-choice question. Circle the letter of your choice.

1. Process of measuring the forward protrusion of the eye.
a. gonioscopy
b. keratometry
c. exophthalmometry
d. tonometry

2. Process of measuring the cornea.
a. gonioscopy
b. keratometry
c. exophthalmometry
d. tonometry

3. Used to identify changes in the blood vessels in the eye and to diagnose systemic diseases.
a. exophthalmometry
b. gonioscopy
c. ophthalmoscopy
d. tonometry

4. Process of measuring the intraocular pressure of the eye.
a. exophthalmometry
b. gonioscopy
c. ophthalmoscopy
d. tonometry

5. Process used to measure the acuteness or sharpness of vision.
a. color vision tests
b. ultrasonography
c. tonometry
d. visual acuity

Abbreviations

Place the correct word, phrase, or abbreviation in the space provided.

1. accommodation ______________________________

2. EM ______________________________

3. Hy ______________________________

4. intraocular lens ______________________________

5. esotropia ______________________________

6. MY ______________________________

7. VA ______________________________

8. IOP ______________________________

9. retrolental fibroplasia ______________________________

10. XT ______________________________

Practical Application

Medical Record Analysis

This exercise contains information, abbreviations, and medical terminology from an actual medical record or case study that has been adapted for this text. The names and any personal information have been created by the author. Read and study each form or case study and then answer the questions that follow. You may refer to Appendix III, *Abbreviations and Symbols*.

INSTRUCTIONS FOR OUTPATIENT CATARACT SURGERY

Task Edit View Time Scale Options Help Date: 17 July 2017

Before Surgery

1. Your surgery has been scheduled for Tuesday, August 2, 2017, as an outpatient at: Dewdrop Surgery Center.
2. Report to the center the day of surgery at 7:10 A.M.
3. The afternoon before surgery and the morning of surgery, use the antibiotics Vigamox and Zymar drops in the right eye to help prevent a bacterial infection. Afternoon and evening before surgery, 1 drop at 3:00, 5:00, 7:00, and 9:00 P.M.
4. Do not eat or drink anything the morning of surgery, except a sip of water to take your medications.
5. Do not wear makeup, fingernail polish, or jewelry to the center.
6. If you are normally taking any medications in the morning, especially heart or blood pressure medications, be sure to take them before you come to the center for surgery. However, if you take insulin or diabetes medication, do not take it until you get home from surgery.
7. Go by the outpatient surgery department at Dewdrop Surgery Center to pre-admit any time before the day of surgery.

After Surgery

1. You may go home shortly after surgery. Be sure to bring someone to drive you home. You may resume normal activities but do not engage in vigorous exercise on the day of surgery. Be careful not to have a fall.
2. The shield may be removed 6 hours after surgery. **DO NOT PUT ANY PRESSURE ON YOUR EYE AND DO NOT RUB YOUR EYE**. Put the Vigamox/Zymar drops in 3 times before you go to bed.
3. Return to Dr. Cedric Emmanuel's office on Wednesday, August 3, 2017, at 10:25 A.M. and further instructions will be given. Bring all your eyedrops to the office with you.
4. Continue any medications that you are taking unless otherwise instructed. Resume your usual diet.
5. If you have mild pain, take Tylenol regular-strength (325 mg) acetaminophen: two tablets every 4–6 hours as needed, not to exceed 12 tablets in 24 hours. If the pain is severe call Dr. Cedric Emmanuel: Office & beeper (123) 456-7890.

Medical Record Questions

Place the correct answer in the space provided.

1. What type of medication is Vigamox and why is it ordered for this patient? ______________________

2. What type of medication is Zymar and why is it ordered for this patient? ______________________

3. Should the patient take his or her heart and blood pressure medicine the morning of surgery? __________ ______________________

4. When should the patient go by the Dewdrop Surgery Center to pre-admit? ______________________

5. If the patient has mild pain, what should he or she take? ______________________

Study and Review I

Anatomy and Physiology

Write your answers to the following questions.

1. List the primary and accessory sex organs of the female reproductive system.

a. ______________________ **b.** ______________________

c. ______________________ **d.** ______________________

e. ______________________ **f.** ______________________

2. The normal position of the uterus is known as ______________________.

3. Define fundus.____.

4. Name the three layers of the uterine wall.

a. ______________________ **b.** ______________________

c. ______________________

5. State two primary functions associated with the uterus.

a. ____

b. ____

6. Define the following terms.

a. Retroflexion ____

____

b. Anteversion ____

____

c. Retroversion ____

____

7. The fallopian tubes are also called the ______________________ ______________________ or ______________________.

8. Should the ovum become impregnated by a spermatozoon while in the fallopian tube, the process of ______________________ occurs.

9. State the two functions of the ovary.

a. ______________________ **b.** ______________________

10. State the three functions of the vagina.

a. ______________________ **b.** ______________________

c. ______________________

11. The breasts or ________________ ______________ are compound alveolar structures.

12. The ______________ is the dark pigmented area found in the skin over each breast, and the ______________ is the elevated area in its center.

13. Define colostrum. ____

____

14. Name the three phases of the menstrual cycle.

a. ______________________ **b.** ______________________

c. ______________________

Overview of Obstetrics

Write your answers to the following questions.

1. ________________ is the branch of medicine that pertains to the care of women during pregnancy, childbirth, and the postpartum period.

2. ________________ is the process in which a sperm penetrates an ovum.

3. The fertilized ovum is also known as a ________________.

4. As the blastocyst develops, it forms a structure with two cavities, the ________________ and ________________.

5. Pregnancy is divided into four stages. Describe each of these stages.

a. Prenatal stage ______________________________________

b. Labor ______________________________________

c. Parturition ______________________________________

d. Postpartum period ______________________________________

6. Labor is divided into three stages. Describe each of these stages.

a. First stage ______________________________

b. Second stage ______________________________

c. Third stage ______________________________

ANATOMY LABELING

Identify the structures shown below by filling in the blanks.

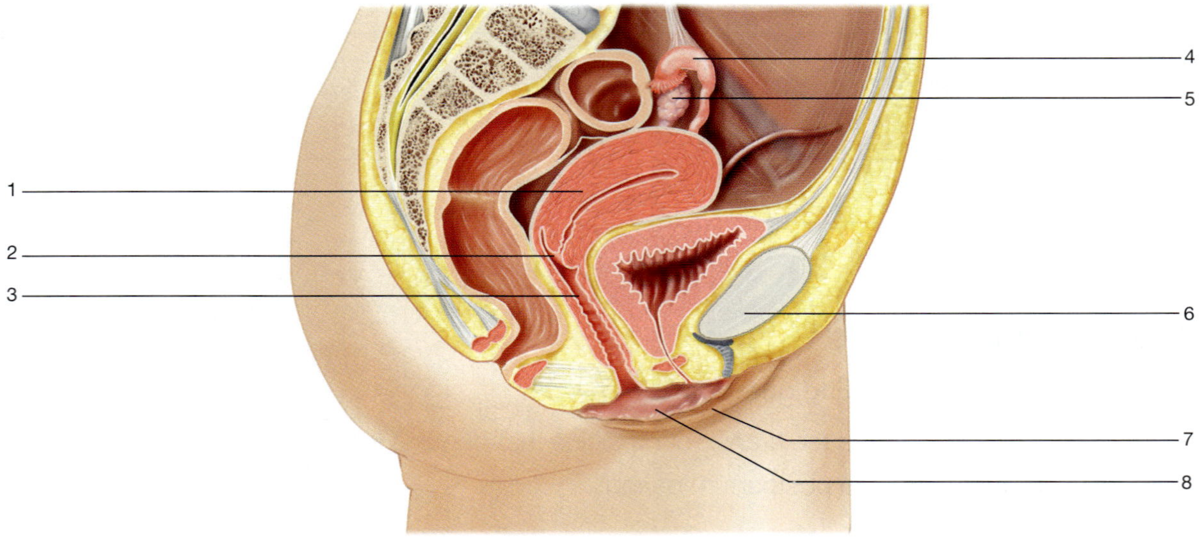

Study and Review II

Word Parts

Prefixes

Give the definitions of the following prefixes.

1. a- ____________________
2. contra- ____________________
3. dys- ____________________
4. ec- ____________________
5. endo- ____________________
6. intra- ____________________
7. oligo- ____________________
8. peri- ____________________
9. post- ____________________
10. retro- ____________________
11. pre- ____________________

Combining Forms

Give the definitions of the following combining forms.

1. abort/o ____________________
2. cervic/o ____________________
3. coit/o ____________________
4. colp/o ____________________
5. culd/o ____________________
6. cyst/o ____________________
7. fibr/o ____________________
8. gynec/o ____________________
9. hyster/o ____________________
10. mamm/o ____________________
11. mast/o ____________________
12. men/o ____________________
13. metr/o ____________________
14. my/o ____________________
15. o/o ____________________
16. oophor/o ____________________
17. pareun/o ____________________
18. rect/o ____________________
19. salping/o ____________________
20. uter/o ____________________
21. vagin/o ____________________
22. vers/o ____________________

Suffixes

Give the definitions of the following suffixes.

1. -al ____________________
2. -arche ____________________
3. -cele ____________________
4. -centesis ____________________
5. -ectomy ____________________
6. -genesis ____________________
7. -ia ____________________
8. -ine ____________________
9. -ion ____________________
10. -ist ____________________
11. -itis ____________________
12. -oma ____________________
13. -osis ____________________
14. -plasty ____________________
15. -rrhagia ____________________
16. -rrhea ____________________
17. -scope ____________________
18. -oid ____________________

Identifying Medical Terms

In the spaces provided, write the medical terms for the following meanings.

1. ____________________ Inflammation of the uterine cervix
2. ____________________ Difficult or painful monthly flow
3. ____________________ Fibrous tissue tumor
4. ____________________ Study of the female
5. ____________________ Surgical excision of the hymen
6. ____________________ Surgical repair of the breast
7. ____________________ Normal monthly flow
8. ____________________ Formation of the ovum
9. ____________________ Difficult or painful sexual intercourse
10. ____________________ Male or female reproductive organs

Matching

Select the appropriate lettered meaning for each of the following words.

_______ 1. laser ablation
_______ 2. lumpectomy
_______ 3. menarche
_______ 4. mittelschmerz
_______ 5. ovulation
_______ 6. gynecologist
_______ 7. contraception
_______ 8. perimenopause
_______ 9. hysterotomy
_______ 10. rectovaginal

a. Beginning of the first monthly flow (menses, menstruation)
b. Surgical removal of a tumor from the breast
c. Abdominal pain that occurs midway between the menstrual periods at ovulation
d. Process in which an ovum is discharged from the cortex of the ovary
e. Procedure that uses a laser to destroy the uterine lining
f. Pertaining to the rectum and vagina
g. Period of gradual changes that lead into menopause
h. Physician who specializes in the study of the female
i. Incision into the uterus
j. Process of preventing conception
k. Lack of monthly flow (menses, menstruation)

Medical Case Snapshots

This learning activity provides an opportunity to relate the medical terminology you are learning to a precise patient case presentation. In the spaces provided, write in your answers.

Case 1

A pregnant 36-year-old woman calls her obstetrician's office, stating, "I am passing bright-red blood and I am cramping. Please tell me what to do. I don't want to lose my baby." The woman was advised to immediately come to the doctor's office. A threatened abortion is one with _______ bleeding or spotting accompanied by _______ or low-back pain. The _______ is not dilated.

Case 2

A 21-year-old female is seen in the emergency room. She has missed her last two periods and feels sick. An ultrasound is ordered stat (immediately). The ultrasound confirmed an _______ pregnancy or tubal _______. An _______ or physician specializing in the care of women during pregnancy, child-birth, and the postpartum period is notified of this patient's condition.

Case 3

A 52-year-old female complains of irregular periods (menses), hot flashes, insomnia, difficult or painful sexual intercourse, and moodiness. The medical term for painful sexual intercourse is ________________. Her condition is known as ________________ (or period of gradual changes that lead into menopause).

Study and Review III

Building Medical Terms

Using the following word parts, fill in the blanks to build the correct medical terms.

bartholin	salping	-genesis
hyster	-al	-pause
mast	-centesis	
men/o	-ectomy	

Definition	Medical Term
1. Inflammation of the Bartholin glands	___________itis
2. Surgical puncture of the cul-de-sac for removal of fluid	culdo__________
3. Surgical excision of the uterus	_______ectomy
4. Surgical removal of a tumor from the breast	lump _________
5. Surgical excision of the breast	________ectomy
6. Cessation of the monthly flow	meno__________
7. Normal monthly flow (menses, menstruation)	_________rrhea
8. Formation of the ovum	oo____________
9. Inflammation of a fallopian tube	___________itis
10. Pertaining to after sexual intercourse	postcoit ________

Combining Form Challenge

Using the combining forms provided, write the medical term correctly.

cervic/o	cyst/o	genital/o
colp/o	fibr/o	gynec/o

1. Inflammation of the uterine cervix: ___________ itis

2. Medical instrument used to examine the vagina and cervix: ___________scope

3. Hernia of the bladder that protrudes into the vagina: _________cele

4. Fibrous tissue tumor: _________ oma

5. Male or female reproductive organs: _________ ia

6. Study of the female, especially the diseases of the female reproductive organs and the breast: ________ logy

Select the Right Term

Select the correct answer, and write it on the line provided.

1. Accessory parts of a structure are ______________.

   abortion | incomplete | adnexa | estrogens

2. Difficult or painful monthly flow (menses or menstruation) is ______________.

   amenorrhea | dysmenorrhea | dyspareunia | eclampsia

3. Refers to any pregnancy, regardless of duration, including the present one is ______________.

   gravida | nulligravida | primigravida | multigravida

4. Vaginal discharge occurring after childbirth is ______________.

   menarche | mittelschmerz | lochia | menorrhagia

5. Serious complication of pregnancy characterized by increasing hypertension, proteinuria, and edema is ______________.

   eclampsia | preeclampsia | placenta previa | endometriosis

6. Process of being turned backward is ______________.

   rectovaginal | toxic shock | retroversion | retroverion

Diagnostic and Laboratory Tests

Select the best answer to each multiple-choice question. Circle the letter of your choice.

1. X-ray of the uterus and fallopian tubes after the injection of a radiopaque substance.
   a. hysterosalpingography
   b. laparoscopy
   c. culdoscopy
   d. mammography

2. Used to examine the ovaries and fallopian tubes.
   a. colposcopy
   b. culdoscopy
   c. laparoscopy
   d. mammography

3. Process of obtaining pictures of the breast by use of x-rays.
   a. colposcopy
   b. culdoscopy
   c. laparoscopy
   d. mammography

4. Screening technique to aid in the detection of cervical/uterine cancer and cancer precursors.
   a. colposcopy
   b. Papanicolaou (Pap) smear
   c. estrogens
   d. mammography

5. Urine test that determines menstrual disorders or possible abortion.
   a. wet mount or wet prep
   b. culdoscopy
   c. Pap smear
   d. pregnanediol

Abbreviations

Place the correct word, phrase, or abbreviation in the space provided.

1. AB ______________________________
2. FHB ______________________________
3. combined oral contraceptives ______________________________
4. intrauterine device ______________________________
5. pelvic inflammatory disease ______________________________
6. cervical intraepithelial neoplasia ______________________________
7. DUB ______________________________
8. PMS ______________________________
9. dilation and curettage ______________________________
10. toxic shock syndrome ______________________________

Practical Application

Soap: Chart Note Analysis

This exercise will make you aware of information, abbreviations, and medical terminology typically found in a gynecology patient's chart note. The names and any personal information have been created by the author. Read and study each form or case study and then answer the questions that follow. You may refer to Appendix III, *Abbreviations and Symbols*.

Task Edit View Time Scale Options Help Date: 17 May 2017

Patient: Smith, Ann M. **Date:** 2/21/17

DOB: 01/24/1969 **Age:** 48 **Gender:** Female

Allergies: Penicillin

S

Subjective:

48 y/o white female presents with complaints of irregular periods, hot flashes, and trouble sleeping. She states, "Sex with my husband has become uncomfortable and I am very moody. I am really having trouble with hot flashes. I wake up in the middle of the night soaked—especially my hair and neck." When asked about her children, she indicates that she has two children, one daughter who is an English teacher and one son who is a pharmacist. She also states that she has never had an abortion. Her LMP was 11/21/16.

O

Objective:

Vital Signs: T: 98.8 F; **P:** 70; **R:** 16; **BP:** 120/78
Ht: 5′ 3″
Wt: 135 lb

General Appearance: Attractive, well groomed, and pleasant. Noted a slight nervousness and concern during initial interview.

GYN:

Breasts: Symmetrical, no palpable masses or tenderness, no dimpling or skin changes

External genitalia: No lesions or inflammation, normal hair distribution with thinning

Cervix: Pink, smooth, no cervical motion tenderness; Pap smear performed

Adnexa uteri: Nontender, no masses

Uterus: NSSC, noted retroversion position, firm, slightly enlarged, with possible uterine fibroid tumor

Rectal exam: No fissures, hemorrhoids, or skin lesions in perianal area. Sphincter tone good, no prolapse. No masses or tenderness.

Pregnancies: gravida 2 para 2 abortions 0

A

Assessment:
Perimenopause

P

Plan: Patient elected the nonprescription treatment for 6 months. To be reevaluated August 2017.

1. Schedule mammogram ASAP. If WNL, then annually.
2. Advised to use over-the-counter (OTC) water-soluble vaginal lubricant for intercourse and moisturizer for vaginal dryness.
3. Advised to go to the laboratory for CBC, cholesterol, triglycerides, and glucose. Check TSH, FSH, and estradiol levels to rule out (R/O) thyroid disorder and obtain hormone baseline levels.
4. Recommended she take a multivitamin and mineral complex that contains 400 mcg of folic acid. Also, take 1500 mg of calcium with vitamin D daily and an antioxidant.
5. Schedule a pelvic ultrasound to R/O uterine fibroid tumor, ASAP.
6. Recommend a bone density study before reevaluation in August.

Chart Note Questions

Place the correct answer in the space provided.

1. What is the abbreviation for gynecology? ______________________
2. What does the statement, "I wake up in the middle of the night soaked—especially my hair and neck," indicate? ______________________
3. What is the medical word for difficult or painful sexual intercourse? ______________________
4. What does gravida 2 indicate? ______________________
5. Why is a pelvic ultrasound recommended? ______________________

Study and Review I

Anatomy and Physiology

Write your answers to the following questions.

1. List the primary and accessory glands of the male reproductive system.

   a. ______________________ b. ______________________

   c. ______________________ d. ______________________

   e. ______________________ f. ______________________

2. Name the supporting structure and accessory sex organs of the male reproductive system.

   a. ______________________ b. ______________________

3. State the vital function of the male reproductive system. ______________________

4. The ______________________ ______________________ is the cone-shaped head of the penis.

5. Define prepuce. ______________________

6. Define smegma. ______________________

7. State two functions of the penis.

   a. ______________________ b. ______________________

8. ______________________ ______________________ is the site of the development of spermatozoa.

9. List five effects of testosterone regarding male development.

   a. ______________________ b. ______________________

   c. ______________________ d. ______________________

   e. ______________________

10. State two functions of the epididymis.

    a. ______________________ b. ______________________

11. The excretory duct of the testes is known by two names, ______________________ ______________________ or ______________________ ______________________.

12. State the function of the seminal vesicles. ______________________________

13. Describe the prostate gland. ______________________________

____

14. Define the condition known as benign prostatic hyperplasia. ______________________________

____

15. The two small pea-sized glands located below the prostate and on either side of the urethra are known as the ______________________ glands or as ______________________ glands.

16. Name the three sections of the male urethra.

a. ______________________________ **b.** ______________________________

c. ______________________________

17. State a function of the male urethra. ______________________________

18. The male urethra is approximately ______________________________ cm long.

Study and Review II

Word Parts

Prefixes

Give the definitions of the following prefixes.

1. a- ______________________
2. an- ______________________
3. circum- ______________________
4. epi- ______________________
5. hydro- ______________________
6. hypo- ______________________
7. oligo- ______________________
8. par- ______________________
9. in- ______________________
10. hetero- ______________________
11. homo- ______________________

Combining Forms

Give the definitions of the following combining forms.

1. balan/o ______________________
2. cis/o ______________________
3. crypt/o ______________________
4. didym/o ______________________
5. ejaculat/o ______________________
6. gon/o ______________________
7. gynec/o ______________________
8. mast/o ______________________
9. mit/o ______________________
10. orch/o ______________________
11. orchid/o ______________________
12. prostat/o ______________________
13. sperm/o ______________________
14. spermat/o ______________________
15. testicul/o ______________________
16. varic/o ______________________
17. vas/o ______________________
18. vesicul/o ______________________
19. zo/o ______________________

Suffixes

Give the definitions of the following suffixes.

1. -al ______________________ **2.** -ar ______________________

3. -cele ______________________ **4.** -cide ______________________

5. -ectomy ______________________ **6.** -genesis ______________________

7. -ia ______________________ **8.** -ion ______________________

9. -ism ______________________ **10.** -itis ______________________

11. -ate ______________________ **12.** -osis ______________________

13. -rrhea ______________________ **14.** -tomy ______________________

Identifying Medical Terms

In the spaces provided, write the medical terms for the following meanings.

1. ______________________ Inflammation of the glans penis

2. ______________________ Surgical excision of the epididymis

3. ______________________ Surgical excision of a testicle

4. ______________________ Foreskin over the glans penis

5. ______________________ Accumulation of fluid in a saclike cavity

6. ______________________ Wartlike growth on the skin

7. ______________________ Sperm germ cell

8. ______________________ Male sex cell

9. ______________________ Agent that kills sperm

10. ______________________ Pertaining to a testicle

Matching

Select the appropriate lettered meaning for each of the following words.

_______ 1. circumcision
_______ 2. coitus
_______ 3. condom
_______ 4. gamete
_______ 5. orchiditis
_______ 6. gonorrhea
_______ 7. infertility
_______ 8. prepuce
_______ 9. spermicide
_______ 10. parenchyma

a. Agent that kills sperm
b. Mature reproductive cell of the male or female
c. Sexual intercourse between a man and a woman
d. Essential cells of a gland or organ that are involved with its function
e. Surgical procedure of removing the foreskin of the penis
f. Thin, flexible protective sheath worn over the penis during copulation to help prevent impregnation or sexually transmitted infection
g. Inflammation of a testicle
h. Inability to produce a viable offspring
i. Causes purulent urethral discharge in the male and purulent vaginal discharge in the female
j. Caused by the bacterium *Chlamydia trachomatis*
k. The foreskin over the glans penis in the male

Medical Case Snapshots

This learning activity provides an opportunity to relate the medical terminology you are learning to a precise patient case presentation. In the spaces provided, write in your answers.

Case 1

A 45-year-old male presents with an inability to achieve and maintain penile erection sufficient to complete satisfactory intercourse. This condition is known as _______ _______. There are many treatment options for ED, with the most popular being drug therapy (see *Drug Highlights*).

Case 2

During the assessment of the newborn male it was noted that the urethra opened on the underside of the penis. This condition is referred to as _______ and an abnormal direction of urine spray is common. In this case, _______ is not recommended for the baby as the foreskin should be kept for use in a surgical repair. Urologists usually recommend repair before the child is _______ months of age.

Case 3

A 60-year-old male complains of difficulty with urinating, "I tend to urinate more frequently, especially at night." This is called ____________. "I feel this sudden need to urinate." This is known as ____________. "Then I have trouble starting my stream." After a complete physical and a digital rectal exam (DRE), the diagnosis was confirmed to be BPH also known as benign ____________ ____________. BPH can also be referred to as having ____________, (which is any condition of the prostate gland that interferes with the flow of urine from the bladder).

Study and Review III

Building Medical Terms

Using the following word parts, fill in the blanks to build the correct medical terms.

hydro-	testicul	-itis
par-	-ate	-genesis
prostat	-cide	
spermat/o	-cele	

Definition	Medical Term
1. Removal of the testicles in a man or ovaries in a woman	castr__________
2. Accumulation of fluid in a saclike cavity	__________cele
3. Inflammation of a testicle	orchid________
4. Essential cells of a gland that are involved with its function	______enchyma
5. Inflammation of the prostate	___________itis
6. Formation of spermatozoa	spermato______

Definition	Medical Term
7. Male sex cell	__________zoon
8. Agent that kills sperm	spermi________
9. Pertaining to a testicle	____________ar
10. Enlargement and twisting of the veins of the spermatic cord	varico_________

Combining Form Challenge

Using the combining forms provided, write the medical term correctly.

balan/o	orchid/o	prostat/o
gon/o	mit/o	vesicul/o

1. Inflammation of the glans penis: ___________itis

2. Highly contagious sexually transmitted infection of the genital mucous membrane: ___________rrhea

3. Incision into a testicle: ___________tomy

4. Ordinary condition of cell division: ___________osis

5. Surgical excision of the prostate: ___________ectomy

6. Inflammation of a seminal vesicle: ___________itis

Select the Right Term

Select the correct answer, and write it on the line provided.

1. Condition in which there is a lack of one or both testes is ___________.

aspermia **anorchism** **azoospermia** **testicular**

2. Surgical procedure of removing the foreskin of the penis is ___________.

condyloma **coitus** **circumcision** **castrate**

3. Condition in which one or both testes fail to descend into the scrotum is ___________.

cryptorchidism **epispadias** **hydrocele** **cryptochidism**

4. Pertains to the same sex is ___________.

eugenics **gamete** **homosexual** **phimosis**

5. Surgical procedure in which the vas deferens are cut, then tied or sealed to prevent the transport of sperm out of the testes, is ___________.

vasectomy **vasotomy** **vesiculitis** **orchidectomy**

6. Sexually transmitted infection caused by *treponema pallidum* is ___________.

herpes **chlamydia** **gonorrhea** **syphilis**

Diagnostic and Laboratory Tests

Select the best answer to each multiple-choice question. Circle the letter of your choice.

1. Test performed on blood serum to detect syphilis.

a. paternity
b. semen
c. FTA-ABS
d. HSV-2

2. Test to determine whether a certain man is the father of a specific child.

a. paternity
b. semen
c. FTA-ABS
d. HSV-2

3. Increased level indicates prostate disease or possibly prostate cancer.

a. fluorescent treponemal antibody
b. prostate-specific antigen
c. semen
d. VDRL

4. Used to determine infertility in men.

a. paternity
b. prostate-specific antigen
c. semen
d. VDRL

5. Increased level can indicate benign prostatic hyperplasia.

a. fluorescent treponemal antibody
b. prostate-specific antigen
c. VDRL
d. venereal disease research laboratory

Abbreviations

Place the correct word, phrase, or abbreviation in the space provided.

1. benign prostatic hyperplasia ______________________

2. GC ______________________

3. human papillomavirus ______________________

4. HSV-2 ______________________

5. STIs ______________________

6. erectile dysfunction ______________________

7. TURP ______________________

8. NGU ______________________

9. venereal disease research laboratory ______________________

10. prostate-specific antigen ______________________

Practical Application

CDC Study

Read the adapted CDC study and then answer the questions that follow.

CDC STUDY FINDS U.S. HERPES RATES REMAIN HIGH

Task Edit View Time Scale Options Help Date: 17 May 2017

1 in 6 Americans Infected; Highest Prevalence among Women and African Americans

About 1 in 6 Americans (16.2%) between the ages of 14 and 49 is infected with herpes simplex virus type 2 (HSV-2), according to the Centers for Disease Control and Prevention. HSV-2 is a lifelong and incurable infection that can cause recurrent and painful genital sores. It remains one of the most common sexually transmitted infections (STIs) in the United States. Research shows that people with herpes are two to three times more likely to acquire HIV, and that herpes can also make HIV-infected individuals more likely to transmit HIV to others. The CDC estimates that over 80% of those with HSV-2 are unaware of their infection. Symptoms may be absent, mild, or mistaken for another condition. And people with HSV-2 can transmit the virus even when they have no visible sores or other symptoms.

"Many individuals are transmitting herpes to others without even knowing it," said John M. Douglas, Jr., M.D., director of CDC's Division of STD Prevention. "We can't afford to be complacent about this disease. It is important that persons with symptoms suggestive of herpes—especially recurrent sores in the genital area—seek clinical care to determine if these symptoms may be due to herpes and might benefit from treatment."

Combination of Prevention Approaches Needed to Reduce National Herpes Rates

Although HSV-2 infection is not curable, there are effective medications available to treat symptoms and prevent outbreaks. Those with known herpes infection should avoid sex when herpes symptoms or sores are present and understand that HSV-2 can still be transmitted when sores are not present. Effective strategies to reduce the risk of HSV-2 infection include abstaining from sexual contact, using condoms consistently and correctly, and limiting the number of sex partners.

CDC Study Questions

Place the correct answer in the space provided.

1. ________________________________ remains one of the most common sexually transmitted infections (STIs) in the United States.

2. About one in six Americans (16.2%) between the ages of __________ and __________ is infected with herpes simplex virus type 2 (HSV-2).

3. Is herpes a lifelong and incurable infection that can cause recurrent and painful genital sores?

   ____

4. The CDC estimates that over ____________________________ percent of those with HSV-2 are unaware of their infection.

5. People with HSV-2 can transmit the virus even when they have no ______________ sores or other symptoms.

Study and Review I

Overview of Oncology

Write your answers to the following questions.

1. Name the three main classifications of cancer.

a. ______________________ **b.** ______________________

c. ______________________

2. Define cell differentiation. ____

____

3. Define dedifferentiation. ____

____

4. Name three ways that malignant cells spread to body parts.

a. ______________________ **b.** ______________________

c. ______________________

5. List the seven warning signals for cancer.

a. ______________________ **b.** ______________________

c. ______________________ **d.** ______________________

e. ______________________ **f.** ______________________

g. ______________________

6. Name four methods used in the treatment of cancer.

a. ______________________ **b.** ______________________

c. ______________________ **d.** ______________________

Study and Review II

Word Parts

Prefixes

Give the definitions of the following prefixes.

1. ana- ______________________
2. astro- ______________________
3. hyper- ______________________
4. neo- ______________________
5. oligo- ______________________
6. pre- ______________________
7. en- ______________________
8. in- ______________________
9. meta- ______________________
10. brachy- ______________________

Combining Forms

Give the definitions of the following combining forms.

1. cancer/o ______________________
2. capsul/o ______________________
3. carcin/o ______________________
4. chori/o ______________________
5. dendr/o ______________________
6. filtrat/o ______________________
7. gli/o ______________________
8. immun/o ______________________
9. lei/o ______________________
10. malign/o ______________________
11. melan/o ______________________
12. mucos/o ______________________
13. mutat/o ______________________
14. myc/o ______________________
15. myel/o ______________________
16. onc/o ______________________
17. palliat/o ______________________
18. remiss/o ______________________
19. reticul/o ______________________
20. rhabd/o ______________________
21. suppress/o ______________________
22. terat/o ______________________
23. tox/o ______________________
24. vir/o ______________________

Suffixes

Give the definitions of the following suffixes.

1. -blast ______
2. -emia ______
3. -gen ______
4. -genes ______
5. -genic ______
6. -ia ______
7. -in ______
8. -itis ______
9. -oma ______
10. -ous ______
11. -plakia ______
12. -plasia ______
13. -plasm ______
14. -ate(d) ______
15. -therapy ______
16. -us ______
17. -al ______
18. -ar ______
19. -ion ______
20. -ive ______
21. -ant ______
22. -stasis ______
23. -oid ______

Identifying Medical Terms

In the spaces provided, write the medical terms for the following meanings.

1. ______ Agent or substance that incites or produces cancer
2. ______ Cancerous tumor derived from cartilage cells
3. ______ Cancerous tumor of the brain
4. ______ Cancerous tumor of smooth muscle tissue
5. ______ Cancer of the blood characterized by overproduction of leukocytes
6. ______ Cancerous tumor of lymphoid tissue
7. ______ Literally means *a black tumor*
8. ______ Cancerous tumor of muscle tissue
9. ______ Cancerous tumor of the kidney occurring mainly in children
10. ______ Cancerous tumor arising in connective tissue

Matching

Select the appropriate lettered meaning for each of the following words.

_______ 1. Hodgkin disease
_______ 2. exacerbation
_______ 3. differentiation
_______ 4. in situ
_______ 5. encapsulated
_______ 6. photodynamic therapy
_______ 7. fungating
_______ 8. hyperplasia
_______ 9. Kaposi sarcoma
_______ 10. metastasis

a. Spreading process of cancer from a primary site to a secondary site
b. Excessive formation and growth of normal cells
c. Enclosed within a sheath
d. Process by which normal cells have a distinct appearance and specialized function
e. Form of lymphoma that occurs in young adults
f. Type of laser therapy that involves the use of a special chemical that is injected into the bloodstream and absorbed by cells all over the body
g. Enclosed within a site, sheath, or capsule
h. Malignant neoplasm that causes violaceous (purplish discoloration), vascular lesions, and general lymphadenopathy
i. Process of increasing the severity of symptoms
j. Process of growing rapidly
k. Agent that causes a change in the genetic structure of an organism

Medical Case Snapshots

This learning activity provides an opportunity to relate the medical terminology you are learning to a precise patient case presentation. In the spaces provided, write in your answers.

Case 1

A 45-year-old female is diagnosed with ductal carcinoma in situ (abbreviated as _______) of the right breast. This type of cancer is confined to the _______ or milk-producing glands or ducts and has not invaded nearby breast tissue. The patient is in stage I. The _______ is smaller than or equal to 2 centimeters in diameter and the _______ lymph nodes test _______ for cancer.

Case 2

A 29-year-old male presents stating, "I was taking a shower and washing my genitals when I found a lump in my right testicle." Upon examination it was noted that the right testicle was firm with a nontender, oval, pea-sized mass that did not reduce with patient lying down. The patient was suspected of having _______ _______, which is a disease in which malignant cells form in the tissues of one or both testicles. To confirm the diagnosis several procedures and tests were ordered. The biopsy was positive for a ___________, a cancerous tumor of the testis.

Case 3

A 70-year-old female presents with a cough that has not gone away. She states that in the last 3 months the cough has gotten worse. She is a smoker, with a history of a pack-a-day for over 35 years. A ___________ cytology (the microscopic examination of cells obtained from a deep-cough sample of mucus in the lungs) is ordered. To confirm the presence of lung cancer, the doctor must perform a ___________ in order to examine tissue from the lung.

Study and Review III

Building Medical Terms

Using the following word parts, fill in the blanks to build the correct medical terms.

lymph	terat	-oma
melan	-plasia	-us
onc/o	-plasm	
remiss	-ive	

Definition	Medical Term
1. Excessive formation and growth of normal cells	hyper_________
2. Cancerous tumor of lymphoid tissue	_________oma
3. Literally means *a cancerous black mole or tumor*	_________oma
4. New tissue formed, such as an abnormal growth or tumor	neo_________
5. Cancer-causing genes	_________genes
6. A form of treatment to relieve symptoms without curing	palliat_________
7. Process of lessening the severity of symptoms	_________ion
8. Cancerous tumor of the testes	semin_________
9. Cancerous tumor of the ovary or testicles	_________oma
10. Pertaining to the inability to open the mouth fully	trism_________

Combining Form Challenge

Using the combining forms provided, write the medical term correctly.

carcin/o	leuk/o	myel/o
immun/o	malign/o	sarc/o

1. Agent or substance that incites or produces cancer: __________ gen

2. Treatment of disease by active, passive, or adoptive immunity: __________ therapy

3. Cancer of the blood characterized by overproduction of leukocytes: __________ emia

4. Pertaining to a bad wandering: __________ ant

5. Tumor arising in the hematopoietic portion of the bone marrow: __________ oma

6. Cancerous tumor arising in connective tissue: __________ oma

Select the Right Term

Select the correct answer, and write it on the line provided.

1. Process by which normal cells lose their specialization and become malignant is __________.

   carcinoid **dedifferentiation** **differentiation** **exacerbation**

2. Spreading process of cancer from a primary site to a secondary site is __________.

   invasive **in situ** **metastasis** **mutation**

3. In radiation therapy, refers to the skin area of entry for the radiation is __________.

   primary site **port** **secondary site** **derma-entry**

4. Process of rapid production; growth by multiplying is __________.

   proliferation **exacerbation** **remission** **invasive**

5. Cancerous tumor of the kidney occurring mainly in children is __________.

   Hodgkin disease **Kaposi sarcoma** **neuroblastoma** **Wilms tumor**

6. Condition of dryness of the mouth is __________.

   trismus **stomatitis** **xerostomia** **mucositis**

Abbreviations

Place the correct word, phrase, or abbreviation in the space provided.

1. adenocarcinoma ____________________
2. biopsy ____________________
3. CA ____________________
4. chemo ____________________
5. deoxyribonucleic acid ____________________
6. IRT ____________________
7. human epidermal growth factor receptor–2/neu ____________________
8. ductal carcinoma in situ ____________________
9. BCC ____________________
10. testicular cancer ____________________

Practical Application

Medical Record Analysis

This exercise contains information, abbreviations, and medical terminology from an actual medical record or case study that has been adapted for this text. The names and any personal information have been created by the author. Read and study each form or case study and then answer the questions that follow. You may refer to Appendix III, *Abbreviations and Symbols*.

RIVER CITY PATHOLOGY

Task | Edit | View | Time Scale | Options | Help | Date: 17 May 2017

Paul Nelson, MD, Lab Director
1048 Peachtree Drive, Suite A 1040
Atlanta, GA 30328
(123)456-7890

PATHOLOGY REPORT

Path#: OB07-0000786	Patient: Betsy Parker	8234
Biopsy: 1/18/17	DOB: 2/24/49 Gender: Female	
Received: 1/18/17	Physician: Jackson Lewis, MD	
Reported: 1/19/17		

Diagnosis: Right Shoulder
Basal Cell Carcinoma, Nodular & Infiltrative Type, Margins Free, see description

---

Clinical data: Clinical BCC Check Margins, Suture Marks Superior Margin at 12 O'CLOCK

Specimen site: Right Shoulder-excision

Gross Description:

The specimen is a portion of skin measuring (cm) 2.4 × 1.3 × 0.3

Microscopic Description:

Present within the dermis are aggregates of basaloid cells with hyperchromatic nuclei, scant cytoplasm, and palisading of the peripheral nuclei. This neoplasm has an infiltrative pattern of growth in the submitted specimen. Sections have been taken to show the base and margins and reveal that the neoplastic process appears to be totally excised in these sections.

Paul Nelson, MD

Medical Record Questions

Place the correct answer in the space provided.

1. What is a neoplasm? ____________________
2. What is the meaning of BCC? ____________________
3. Why is it important to indicate "margins free" in the diagnosis? ____________________
4. What was the location of this specimen? ____________________
5. What is the meaning of cm? ____________________

Study and Review I

Overview of Radiology and Nuclear Medicine

Write your answers to the following questions.

1. Define radiology. ______________________________

2. Name three characteristics of x-rays.

   a. ______________________ b. ______________________

   c. ______________________

3. Name two dangers of x-rays.

   a. ______________________ b. ______________________

4. List five safety precautions designed to prevent unnecessary exposure to x-rays.

   a. ______________________ b. ______________________

   c. ______________________ d. ______________________

   e. ______________________

5. Name five techniques used in diagnostic imaging.

   a. ______________________ b. ______________________

   c. ______________________ d. ______________________

   e. ______________________

Study and Review II

Word Parts

Prefixes

Give the definitions of the following prefixes.

1. sub- ______________________
2. intra- ______________________
3. milli- ______________________
4. ultra- ______________________
5. ir- ______________________

Combining Forms

Give the definitions of the following combining forms.

1. act/o ______________________
2. angi/o ______________________
3. arteri/o ______________________
4. arthr/o ______________________
5. bronch/o ______________________
6. cinemat/o ______________________
7. digit/o ______________________
8. ech/o ______________________
9. fluor/o ______________________
10. gen/o ______________________
11. mamm/o ______________________
12. oscill/o ______________________
13. physic/o ______________________
14. pyel/o ______________________
15. radi/o ______________________
16. salping/o ______________________
17. sial/o ______________________
18. son/o ______________________
19. therm/o ______________________
20. tom/o ______________________
21. tract/o ______________________

Suffixes

Give the definitions of the following suffixes.

1. -er ______________________
2. -genic ______________________
3. -al ______________________
4. -gram ______________________
5. -graph ______________________
6. -graphy ______________________
7. -ic ______________________
8. -ion ______________________

9. -ist ____________________

10. -itis ____________________

11. -ive ____________________

12. -logy ____________________

13. -ous ____________________

14. -scope ____________________

15. -scopy ____________________

16. -therapy ____________________

17. -ide ____________________

Identifying Medical Terms

In the spaces provided, write the medical terms for the following meanings.

1. ____________________ A medical imaging technique used to visualize the inside, or lumen, of blood vessels and organs of the body
2. ____________________ Process of making an x-ray record of a joint
3. ____________________ X-ray record of the gallbladder made visible through the use of a radiopaque contrast medium
4. ____________________ A process resulting in the gain or loss of one or more electrons in neutral atoms
5. ____________________ Process of obtaining x-ray pictures of the breast
6. ____________________ 0.001 Ci
7. ____________________ Literally means *one who specializes in nature*
8. ____________________ Process whereby radiant energy is propagated through space or matter
9. ____________________ Characterized by emitting radiant energy
10. ____________________ Person skilled in making x-ray records
11. ____________________ Pertaining to property of permitting the passage of radiant energy
12. ____________________ Pertaining to property of obstructing the passage of radiant energy
13. ____________________ Record produced by ultrasonography

Matching

Select the appropriate lettered meaning for each of the following words.

_____________ **1.** PET scan
_____________ **2.** cathode
_____________ **3.** beam
_____________ **4.** cassette
_____________ **5.** rad
_____________ **6.** lead
_____________ **7.** radium
_____________ **8.** scan
_____________ **9.** shield
_____________ **10.** tagging

a. Protective structure used to prevent or reduce the passage of particles or radiation
b. Radioactive isotope used to treat certain malignant diseases
c. Ray of light
d. Nuclear medicine imaging technique that helps physicians see how the organs and tissues inside the body are actually functioning
e. Negative pole of an electrical current
f. Loss of energy
g. Light-proof case or holder for x-ray film
h. Process of tracing a radioactive isotope that has become involved in metabolic or chemical reactions
i. Process of using a moving device or sweeping beam of radiation to produce images of organs or structures of the body
j. Amount of radiation absorbed
k. Metallic chemical element

Medical Case Snapshot

This learning activity provides an opportunity to relate the medical terminology you are learning to a precise patient case presentation. In the spaces provided, write in your answers.

A 37-year-old female presents stating, "I was doing my monthly breast exam, just after my period, and I felt this lump in my left breast." Also explaining, "It doesn't hurt, but I am afraid that it might be cancer." After a complete evaluation and exam, a mammography was scheduled. The _____________ is the actual x-ray record of the breast. The two types are _____________ and diagnostic. This type of x-ray can detect _____________ in the breast often before a lump can be felt.

Study and Review III

Building Medical Terms

Using the following word parts, fill in the blanks to build the correct medical terms.

myel/o	sial/o	-ion
physic	-gram	-opaque
radi/o	-graphy	

Definition	Medical Term
1. X-ray record of the bronchial tree	broncho______
2. Process of making an x-ray record of the salivary ducts and glands	sialo______
3. Process of obtaining x-ray picture of the breast	mammo______
4. X-ray record of the spinal cord	______gram
5. Literally means *one who specializes in nature*	________ist
6. Process by which radiant energy is propagated through space	radiat____
7. Pertaining to property of permitting passage of radiant energy	____lucent
8. Pertaining to property of obstructing passage of radiant energy	radi____
9. Treatment of disease by the use of radioactive substances	____therapy
10. Process of making an x-ray record of veins	veno___

Combining Form Challenge

Using the combining forms provided, write the medical term correctly.

arthr/o	son/o	tom/o
radi/o	therm/o	

1. Process of making an x-ray record of a joint: __________graphy
2. Treatment of disease by the use of x-rays, radium, and other radioactive substances: __________therapy
3. Picture produced on a sensitized film or plate by rays: __________graph
4. Process of using ultrasound to produce a record of ultrasonic echoes: __________graphy
5. Process of recording heat patterns of the body's surface: __________graphy
6. Process of cutting across and producing images of single tissue planes: __________graphy

Select the Right Term

Select the correct answer, and write it on the line provided.

1. Process of making an x-ray record of the arteries is ______________.

   angiocardiogram **arteriography** **arthrography** **angiography**

2. X-ray record of the gallbladder is ______________.

   cholangiogram **cholecystogram** **choleangiogram** **cholcystogram**

3. Characterized by emitting radiant energy is ______________.

   radionuclide **radium** **radiation** **radioactive**

4. International unit for describing exposure dose of x-ray is ______________.

   radium **rad** **roentgen** **millicurie**

5. Protective structure used to prevent passage of radiation is ______________.

   tagging **shield** **cathode** **rad**

6. Process of using ultrasound to produce a record of ultrasonic echoes is ______________.

   sialography **tomography** **ultrasonography** **ultrasonic**

Abbreviations

Place the correct word, phrase, or abbreviation in the space provided.

1. anteroposterior ______________________________
2. barium ______________________________
3. computed tomography ______________________________
4. IR ______________________________
5. lat ______________________________
6. Ra ______________________________
7. magnetic resonance imaging ______________________________
8. PA ______________________________
9. curie ______________________________
10. PET ______________________________

Practical Application

Medical Record Analysis

This exercise contains information, abbreviations, and medical terminology from an actual medical record or case study that has been adapted for this text. The names and any personal information have been created by the author. Read and study each form or case study and then answer the questions that follow. You may refer to Appendix III, *Abbreviations and Symbols*.

LA VISTA WOMEN'S CENTER

Task Edit View Time Scale Options Help Date: 17 May 2017

7785 West Walnut Drive
Clifton Park, NY 12065-2919
(123) 456-7890

Sarah Jane Justice
2345 Maple Avenue
Clifton Park, NY 12065-2919
Date of Mammogram 5-6-17

We wish to report the following on your mammography examination. A report will be sent to your referring physician or other healthcare provider.

☐ Normal/Negative. No evidence of cancer.

☐ No abnormality seen but comparison with previous mammograms will be performed when and if they can be obtained.

☐ Probably benign (not cancer). Recommended repeat mammogram in 6 months. Please call your physician for an order, then call for appointment at (518) 789-1234.

☐ Additional imaging studies are needed to complete evaluation, such as ultrasound or additional mammographic views. Please call your physician for an order, then call for appointment.

☐ Previous films needed. There is a finding on your mammogram that needs to be compared to previous mammograms.

■ Abnormal. There is a finding on your mammogram that requires further tests for a more thorough evaluation. You should contact your physician or other healthcare provider as soon as possible.

Interpreting Radiologist: Steven Presley Woods, MD

Should you develop a lump or any changes in your breast before your next screening mammogram, contact your physician or other healthcare provider for an exam without delay.

Medical Record Questions

Place the correct answer in the space provided.

1. Define mammography. ______________________________
2. Why is there a box for previous films needed? ______________________________
3. This patient had an abnormal mammogram. What does this indicate? ______________________________
4. What does a normal/negative mammogram indicate? ______________________________
5. Who else is sent a copy of the report? ______________________________

Study and Review I

Overview: Mental Health and Mental Disorders

Write your answers to the following questions.

1. A ______________________________ is an abnormal condition of the brain or mind.

2. List the three mental disorders that are listed among the top 10 causes of disability in the United States.

a. ______________________________ **b.** ______________________________

c. ______________________________

3. ______________________________ is the branch of medicine that deals with the study, diagnosis, and treatment of mental disorders.

4. Give the three basic forms of treatment for mental disorders.

a. ______________________________ **b.** ______________________________

c. ______________________________

5. ______________________________ is a method of obtaining a detailed account of past and present mental and emotional experiences and repressions.

Study and Review II

Word Parts

Prefixes

Give the definitions of the following prefixes.

1. an- ____________________
2. hypo- ____________________
3. para- ____________________
4. pyro- ____________________

Combining Forms

Give the definitions of the following combining forms.

1. agor/a ____________________
2. centr/o ____________________
3. cycl/o ____________________
4. delus/o ____________________
5. neur/o ____________________
6. path/o ____________________
7. phren/o ____________________
8. psych/o ____________________
9. schiz/o ____________________
10. somat/o ____________________
11. thym/o ____________________

Suffixes

Give the definitions of the following suffixes.

1. -form ____________________
2. -ia ____________________
3. -ic ____________________
4. -ion ____________________
5. -ism ____________________
6. -ist ____________________
7. -mania ____________________
8. -noia ____________________
9. -orexia ____________________
10. -osis ____________________
11. -phobia ____________________
12. -therapy ____________________
13. -tic ____________________

Identifying Medical Terms

In the spaces provided, write the medical terms for the following meanings.

1. ______________________ Intense fear and anxiety of any place or situation where escape might be difficult, leading to avoidance of such situations
2. ______________________ Condition in which a person lacks feelings and emotions
3. ______________________ Fixed, false belief or abnormal perception
4. ______________________ Mental disorder marked by altered mood and loss of interest in things that are usually pleasurable
5. ______________________ Pertaining to being self-centered
6. ______________________ Mental disorder characterized by excessive excitement; literally means *madness*
7. ______________________ Morbid and persistent fear of a specific object, activity, or situation that results in a compelling desire to avoid the feared stimulus
8. ______________________ Physician who specializes in the study and treatment of mental disorders
9. ______________________ Method of treating mental disorders by using psychological techniques instead of physical methods
10. ______________________ Literally means *a madness for fire*

Matching

Select the appropriate lettered meaning for each of the following words.

_____________ **1.** dysthymia

_____________ **2.** seasonal affective disorder

_____________ **3.** bipolar disorder

_____________ **4.** schizophrenia

_____________ **5.** delusion

_____________ **6.** hallucination

_____________ **7.** obsessive–compulsive disorder

_____________ **8.** posttraumatic stress disorder

_____________ **9.** generalized anxiety disorder

_____________ **10.** attention-deficit/hyperactivity disorder

a. Mental disorder characterized by positive, negative, and cognitive symptoms

b. Process of experiencing sensations that have no source

c. Brain disorder also known as *manic-depressive illness* that causes unusual shifts in a person's mood, energy, and ability to function

d. Less severe type of depression involving long-term, chronic symptoms that do not disable but keep the person from functioning well or from feeling good

e. Debilitating anxiety disorder that can develop following a terrifying event

f. Characterized by bizarre thoughts that have no basis in reality

g. Form of depression that appears related to fluctuations in a person's exposure to natural light

h. Characterized by much higher levels of anxiety than people normally experience day to day

i. Involves persistent, unwelcome thoughts or images or the urgent need to engage in certain rituals that the person cannot control

j. One of the most common childhood disorders and can continue through adolescence and adulthood

k. Anxiety syndrome and panic disorder

Medical Case Snapshot

This learning activity provides an opportunity to relate the medical terminology you are learning to a precise patient case presentation. In the spaces provided, write in your answers.

A 67-year-old female complains of sadness. She describes loss of interest in eating and social activities.

After careful evaluation and examination, it was determined that this patient was experiencing depression.

This is a ___________ ___________ marked by altered ___________ and loss of interest in things that are usually pleasurable. A less severe type of this condition known as ___________ involves long-term, chronic symptoms.

Study and Review III

Abbreviations

Place the correct word, phrase, or abbreviation in the space provided.

1. cognitive-behavioral therapy ____________________
2. *Diagnostic and Statistical Manual of Mental Disorders*, Fifth Edition ____________________
3. ECT ____________________
4. MMPI-2 ____________________
5. National Institute of Mental Health ____________________
6. OCD ____________________
7. posttraumatic stress disorder ____________________
8. SAD ____________________
9. TAT ____________________
10. World Health Organization ____________________

Practical Application

Medical Record Analysis

This exercise contains information, abbreviations, and medical terminology from an actual medical record or case study that has been adapted for this text. The names and any personal information have been created by the author. Read and study each form or case study and then answer the questions that follow. You may refer to Appendix III, *Abbreviations and Symbols*.

DEPARTMENT OF SOCIAL SERVICES

Task Edit View Time Scale Options Help Date: 19 June 2017

Disability Evaluation Division
1888 Golden Gate Blvd., Suite 10
San Francisco, CA 94132
Re: Rotha, Maly # 123-45-6789

Dear Staff:

Thank you for referring to me the case of Ms. Rotha for psychiatric evaluation. She was examined in psychiatric consultation on June 17, 2017. No physical exam was performed. No psychological testing was given. Medical records provided were reviewed. The patient was a clean, neatly dressed, well-groomed Asian female. She understood English and responded to questions. There was no evidence of any ambulation difficulties or speech impediments. Energy level was described as poor, with description of fatigue with minimal exertion.

History of Present Illness

Ms. Rotha is a 42-year-old Cambodian female. She lives in an apartment with her husband and three children. She describes feeling sick all the time and too weak and tired, dizzy and depressed to do anything except "rest." Currently, she is taking a combination of five different medications under the care of two different physicians. She takes Proventil inhaler for relief of asthmatic symptoms, analgesics, decongestants, and two different forms of tricyclic antidepressants. She feels that the medications are helping her. She is not receiving any formal psychiatric treatment with or without medication.

Mental Examination

There is no evidence or history of alcoholism or illicit drug use. She is oriented to time, place, persons, and events. There is no evidence of delusion or hallucinations at the present time and no history of such in the past. There is no evidence of paranoia such as feelings of being persecuted or plotted against. Thought content is generally well organized, coherent, and relevant without flight of ideas or loose associations.

Depression is manifested by occasional crying, usually occurring every other day. There is fitful sleep. There are occasional nightmares. There is no suicidal ideation or history of any suicide attempts.

(*continued*)

Memory for recent and remote events, she feels, is impaired. She cannot recall her Social Security number. She can recall her address and phone number. She can do simple arithmetic.

Medical Opinion

It is my medical opinion that at Ms. Rotha's current level of daily functioning, she has minimal difficulty in relating to others. In appearance she seems to have the ability to care for her personal needs. How much her interest, habits, and daily activities are constricted as a result of mental impairments is difficult to assess because it is my medical opinion that this represents a factitious disorder, although posttraumatic stress disorder should not be ruled out.

Very truly yours,

Hana Eun Kim, MD

Medical Record Questions

Place the correct answer in the space provided.

1. State the symptoms Ms. Rotha described. ______________________________
2. What medications does this patient take? ______________________________
3. What is a delusion? ______________________________
4. Define hallucination. ______________________________
5. Define factitious disorder. ______________________________